THE CONTRACEPTIVE ETHOS

PHILOSOPHY AND MEDICINE

Editors:

H. TRISTRAM ENGELHARDT, JR.

Center for Ethics, Medicine and Public Issues,
The Baylor College of Medicine, Houston, Texas, U.S.A.

STUART F. SPICKER

University of Connecticut School of Medicine,
Health Center, Farmington, Connecticut, U.S.A.

VOLUME 27

THE CONTRACEPTIVE ETHOS

Reproductive Rights and Responsibilities

Edited by

STUART F. SPICKER

University of Connecticut School of Medicine, Health Center,
Farmington, Connecticut, U.S.A.

WILLIAM B. BONDESON

University of Missouri–Columbia,
Columbia, Missouri, U.S.A.

and

H. TRISTRAM ENGELHARDT, JR.

Center for Ethics, Medicine and Public Issues,
The Baylor College of Medicine,
Houston, Texas, U.S.A.

D. REIDEL PUBLISHING COMPANY

A MEMBER OF THE KLUWER ACADEMIC PUBLISHERS GROUP

DORDRECHT / BOSTON / LANCASTER / TOKYO

Library of Congress Cataloging-in-Publication Data

CIP

The Contraceptive ethos.

   (Philosophy and medicine ; v. 27)
   Based on the Sixteenth Symposium on Philosophy
and Medicine, held at the Health Sciences Center of
the University of Missouri—Columbia on Apr. 21–23,
1983, and sponsored by the Health Care and Human
Values Program of the University of Missouri—
Columbia School of Medicine.
   Includes bibliographies and index.
   1. Birth control—Moral and ethical aspects—
Congresses. 2. Contraception—Moral and ethical
aspects—Congresses. 3. Contraceptives—Congresses.
I. Spicker, Stuart F., 1937–   . II. Bondeson,

William B., 1938–   . III. Engelhardt, H. Tristram
(Hugh Tristram), 1941–   . IV. Symposium on
Philosophy and Medicine (16th : 1983 : University of
Missouri—Columbia Health Science Center)
   V. University of Missouri-Columbia. Health Care and
Human Values Program. VI. Series. [DNLM:
1. Contraception—congresses. 2. Family Planning—
congresses. 3. Public Opinion—congresses. 4. Social
Responsibility—congresses. W3 PH609 v.27 /
HQ 766 C7644 1983]
HQ766.15.C66   1987   176   87-23432
ISBN 1-55608-035-2

Published by D. Reidel Publishing Company
P.O. Box 17, 3300 AA Dordrecht, Holland

Sold and distributed in the U.S.A. and Canada
by Kluwer Academic Publishers,
101 Philip Drive, Norwell, MA 02061, U.S.A.

In all other countries, sold and distributed
by Kluwer Academic Publishers Group,
P.O. Box 322, 3300 AH Dordrecht, Holland

Printed in The Netherlands.

TABLE OF CONTENTS

v

ACKNOWLEDGEMENTS

This volume developed from a symposium directed to the theme 'Reproductive Rights and Responsibilities: Medicine and the New Biology'. This, the Sixteenth Symposium on Philosophy and Medicine, was held at the Health Sciences Center of the University of Missouri – Columbia, on April 21, 22, and 23, 1983. During this period of gestation, much has been altered and some additions have been made. Its final form emerged from discussions between the participants and the authors of essays and commentaries. We gratefully acknowledge the contributions made by many individuals who attended this symposium and who, through their comments and discussions with the authors, enabled them to revise and structure their essays as they now appear in this volume. We wish, in addition, to thank all of those who have assisted us in developing this volume from the proceedings of the symposium. From among the many to whom we are in debt, we would especially like to mention Sarah K. Beckett, J. D., of West Hartford, Professor Emeritus Charlotte H. Clark, Ph.D., of the University of Hartford (Connecticut), and Ms. Jenny Ebstein, who inherited the post-symposium manuscripts. We are grateful to them for their careful reading and constructive suggestions.

We want to express our gratitude to all who helped to make possible the symposium from which this volume grew. We are in debt to the Health Care and Human Values Program of the University of Missouri – Columbia, School of Medicine, who sponsored the symposium. The project was supported by grants from The National Endowment for the Humanities (No. RD–20290–82); The Education and Research Foundation of the American Medical Association; and the Ortho Pharmaceutical Corporation; however, the viewpoints or recommendations expressed in the volume are not necessarily those of the Endowment, the American Medical Association or the Ortho Pharmaceutical Corporation.

The Editors also would like to thank William Bradshaw, M.D., Director of Continuing Education and Extension for the Health Professions (now Dean, School of Medicine); Mr. Weldon Webb, Assistant Director of Continuing Education and Extension for the Health

Professions; Dr. Barbara Uehling, Past-Chancellor of the University of
Missouri – Columbia; Charles Lobeck, M.D., former Dean of the
School of Medicine; Dr. Ronald Bunn, Provost of the University of
Missouri – Columbia; John Davenport, M.D., Assistant Professor of
Neurology; Joseph Lamberti, Associate Professor of Psychiatry; Mr.
William Fisch, Professor of Law; Dr. Joseph J. Bien, Professor and
Chairman, Department of Philosophy; and the members of the Health
Care and Human Values Program Committee.

Special thanks should be given to Mrs. Judy Wilson, Research Assistant in the Health Care and Human Values Program, for her superb
handling of all the administrative details which made the symposium a
success.

To the many individuals who labored unselfishly in the preparation
and conduct of this symposium in philosophy and medicine we are
deeply grateful; by their efforts a symposium came into being that
allowed sustained cross-disciplinary discussion concerning the interrela-
tions of the major secular learned professions.

STUART F. SPICKER
WILLIAM B. BONDESON
H. TRISTRAM ENGELHARDT, JR.

INTRODUCTION

Soon after the symposium of April, 1983, which served to initiate the essays and commentaries included in this volume, the world's attention focussed on the AIDS epidemic and, ironically, millions of persons were (and presently are) urged to return to prophylaxis – especially condoms – to begin to forestall the epidemic known as AIDS, especially since this syndrome is lethal in virtually all cases. We say 'ironically' because the subject of contraception, when approached by the planners of the symposium, was intended to focus attention on the philosophical issue of freedom which advances in contraceptive technology made possible for millions of people throughout the world. Moreover, effective contraception not only liberated persons from unwanted pregnancies, it carried with it new moral responsibilities which are inextricably linked to personal rights in free and open societies; and even if a society is not open or a democratic polity in the broadest sense, contraceptive use is a significant socio-political force which governments could and do manipulate for political and economic ends.

It is commonplace to note in media coverage that the AIDS epidemic has once again initiated debate around the issue of constitutional protection of an individual citizen's sexual privacy. Many are asking whether there is a compelling state interest that warrants government intrusion into the sexual privacy of individuals. Since the courts are not the only venue for the ultimate guardianship of the liberties and welfare of individuals – legislatures also have this mandate – there is grave concern that legislatures as well as courts will act in ways to control public health and safety, and that this will translate into intrusion into and infringement upon personal rights. Hence, the argument runs, even if, at times, promoting morality may be a legitimate state purpose, the essential question is one of government power: How far should state legislatures, presumably representing the views of the majority, regulate the activities of individual citizens?

This volume, *The Contraceptive Ethos: Reproductive Rights and Responsibilities*, it should be clear at the outset, does not address the most broadly cast issues that constitute the ecological crises around the globe;

Stuart F. Spicker, William B. Bondeson, and M. Tristram Engelhardt, Jr.
The Contraceptive Ethos, ix-xxiv.
© 1987 *by D. Reidel Publishing Company.*

it is purposely more finely focussed, as it attends to those problems
which have their roots in medicine and especially biomedical technology
which have, through various forms of laboratory research, provided the
possibility of various forms of contraception, though perhaps none
perfectly satisfies all the criteria demanded by men and women alike; we
want an inexpensive, easy to use, comfortable, reliable, and risk-free
method which does not produce any harmful side effects, and preferably
no side effects at all.

In the November 21, 1985, issue of the *New England Journal of
Medicine*, three professors from Harvard Medical School published the
results of their experiment on the effect of 'Coca-Cola'[R] on sperm
motility. They may, of course, have been simply playing lightly on the
'Coke is it' theme, and everyone should be able to have some fun, even
in prestigious publications. But this experiment was in reality a response
to the rumor that Coca-Cola is said to be used in developing countries
for the express purpose of vaginal, post-coital contraception. Whether
or not this is the case, this brief 'Correspondence' in the nation's leading
medical periodical bears testimony not only to the results – where (by
the way) Diet Coke outperformed Old ('Classic') Coke, New Coke, and
Caffeine-free New Coke by reducing sperm motility to zero at one
minute – but to the increasing interest in spermicidal effects and contraception generally. Apparently, all present and available methods of
contraception fail in one or more ways in achieving the desired ends,
even Diet Coke. This limitation is sometimes called the condition of
'technological ignorance', where one can claim that biomedical technology along with appropriate clinical verification are still in the future. In
short, we are not satisfied that we have achieved the contraceptive
advance toward which we have made great efforts, and toward which
numerous industrial/technological researchers are working.

In addition to technological ignorance, there is of course the matter of
'social ignorance', where the major contraceptive means are still unknown in many parts of the world; and, as the present AIDS epidemic
has made salient, the importance and efficacy of (say) condoms is still
not adequately understood. Moreover, even when contraceptive efficacy and its importance for health maintenance is understood and appreciated, contraceptive devices may be feared for pseudo-medical reasons,
or simply not used due to selfish motives related to pleasure enhance-
ment.

Again, as one can learn from the debate concerning the propriety of advertising AIDS-reducing prophylaxis on network television and radio, even prudishness can serve to limit the dissemination of information. One has only to observe the success of the Chinese and Japanese in their direct and open national campaigns to lower the birth rate to see the power of the media in its display of contraceptive information. Yet prudishness is still powerful in Western nations, and thus the many moralists who firmly believe that it is morally wrong to publicly describe the efficacy and power of prophylaxis are a significant social force, and their influence at the present time is not only not diminishing, it should not be underestimated. Paradoxically, then, just as we were told of our new freedoms due to the newly-derived contraceptive ethos, the AIDS epidemic struck and inhibited individuals even in their use of prophylactic condoms since the only reasonable and effective means, we are told, is the condom. Political groups will surely continue to exert their power, much of which will prove an obstacle to the communication of contraceptive information. Having said this, it is important to note that prudishness is deeply linked to religion, but we must leave this relation unaddressed, for to explore it here risks digressing to the teleology of prophylaxis with regard to the goal of disease prevention, when the theme of the volume demands that contraceptive technology be discussed in the context of numerous reproductive issues, and eventually against the background of population control.

Someone once remarked that 'people are pollution'. This, to be sure, is too vicious and harsh a judgment, though it reflects the anti-human prejudice of a number of ecologists. They have informed us, for example, that during the past decade the world's population has increased from 4 to 4.8 billion people – which is equivalent to adding a population to the globe in numbers approaching that of India's present population. Even if the growth rate decreases from 1.7 to 1.5% a year, as is hopefully projected, 6.1 billion people are expected to inhabit the earth by the year 2000, according to United Nations' figures, made public on August 14, 1984, in the Text of the Declaration by International Population at its Conference in Mexico City, and later adopted by the United Nations International Conference on Population.

The distribution of the world's population, the flexibility of the ecological systems in which various sub-populations thrive or suffer, the nature of nations' social traditions and attitudes, these and other concerns surely play a notable part in determining the degree of ecological destructiveness or its regeneration. However, a careful analysis of these and other ecological forces reveals that a reduction in the rate of population growth alone will not necessarily reduce the extent of population or even the rate of depletion of natural resources around the globe. Thus from the perspective of ecological concerns one cannot be certain of the precise importance of population growth alone.

Although such broadly cast issues are not taken up in this volume, the themes addressed by the contributors do include the social dimensions of contraceptive policy, and hence in Section II geopolitics is introduced by Thomas Halper, who addresses the unexpected consequences of population growth in terms of political leverage; for in some nations reductions in population of particular interest groups or racial groups can lead to a rapid transformation of political power from the hands of the old majority to those who were the previous minority, both in terms of numbers and in terms of political control. But the former majority can become a geopolitical minority which will significantly affect the political base of that nation state. In order not to mislead the reader in thinking that population control has only ecological effects, it is important to address this geopolitical issue, where, for example, a large population group elects to carry out a policy of 'population control' (which usually signals population reduction) by means of a propaganda machine that advocates and even rewards those who practice contraception, and perhaps other forms of population control, e.g., infanticide, abortion, sterilization, periodic abstinence and total continence. We then may come full circle, and advocate the adoption of a contraceptive ethos where legislation is perhaps no longer needed to achieve such reduction.

The authors in this volume tend to address the more concrete implications of the contraceptive ethos by examining the relationship between love and sexual activity *not* directed to procreation, and sexual activity whose end is procreation in the context of family planning.

In short, the contributors to this volume appear to agree (since they all tacitly assume it) that the world's population simply cannot continue to increase at its present rate; to do so would lead to a dramatically overcrowded world where many would be guilty of stealing from the commons, a world in which no one would have sufficient room, and the depletion of resources would be inevitable.

Finally, the contributors to this collection do not accept the thesis that contraception is to be identified either with infanticide, sterilization, or abortion – the latter two means being the most widespread ways of controlling population in the Third World. As they see it, contraception and its various techniques not only tend to inhibit procreation, but the authors tend to agree that the function of the human sex organs is not necessarily directed to procreation. They all reflect the secular view that it is not morally wrong for persons to intervene in the human reproductive process by using various forms of contraception to inhibit further procreation and increased world population. Thus a secular view of contraception and its use is shared even where the authors have expressed their religious persuasion. Apparently there is no intrinsic contradiction between deeply religious convictions and contraceptive advocacy and use. For many religiously committed persons contraception is even morally demanded when civilization is threatened and dangerous population increases risk everyone.

This volume in the *Philosophy and Medicine* series, then, takes as its point of departure not the pending crisis rooted in over-population, but rather the fact that biomedical science will continue to affect individual responsibility in sexual practices, only one goal of which is to regulate family size. There is an ever-growing number of persons who contend that even if parents of large families can afford to raise their children in comfort, they still impose a burden on their neighbors. Selfishness, where it can be discerned, is not yet a virtue. In fact, there is in some societies a growing moral pressure against the parents of large families. This social phenomenon is addressed when we turn our attention to China, where social pressure has led to legislative enactments where a nation state claims the right to propagandize and even to coerce its citizens to have no more than a fixed number of children. Social policy accompanied by political force once again raises the question of just how far, morally, a government should intervene in the reproductive rights of its responsible citizens. What precisely is the role of law when governments move to regulate reproduction and family size? These and many other related questions are addressed by the contributors to this volume.

John T. Noonan opens Section I, drawing on the history of contraceptive techniques and pertinent religious and moral teachings to define the relationship between contraception and its social and moral context.

Noonan believes that the use of contraception (including abortion as a way of limiting births) has always depended as much on the political, religious, moral, or ethical context as it has on the existence or knowledge of particular techniques. For instance, at some times social or governmental pressures for increased births may have been key; at other times, pressures for improving the 'quality of life' have been more important to the society than the quantity of births. In some cultures it has been tremendously important for religious reasons to have at least one male child. During recent historical time, it has been crucial to procreate according to the laws of nature as interpreted by the Catholic Church; respecting 'personhood' of the conceptus has at times been of overarching importance, while the definition of 'person' has, of course, been different from time to time under different doctrines.

Contraceptive techniques have improved tremendously Noonan observes, hoping that with increased sophistication we may have the opportunity to strike a balance among competing values. From the availability of technology we need not proceed directly to its use; rather, by choosing among contraception of different kinds, abortion, or no contraception, we may affirm the values which today are not predetermined by national goals or moral or religious absolutes, as they have been in the past.

James Reed, an historian, provides an extended case history of the manner in which the development of effective contraception has depended upon contemporary cultural determinants – the attitudes toward sexual practices and, most particularly, the place of the female as primarily a home-worker and helper or as a person with a function outside the home and away from children.

Reed argues that while there has always been effective contraception, in America of the 19th century, such information was suppressed in a wave of anxiety over diminished birth rates among the established classes and over the tide of prolific, non-Protestant immigrants. Abortion was also proscribed at this time, though until then it had been tolerated. The cultural environment changed at the turn of the century and some premarital sex became well-established.

Nevertheless, Reed maintains, due to countervailing feelings, no major efforts in our century were made to improve contraception until decades after it was feasible to do so. The history of contraception in this century seems to have been driven by feminists, among them Margaret Sanger, and those physicians who (having monopolized the distribution of contraceptive means) appreciated the hazard and perhaps the futility of suppressing this information and new forms of contraception. By 1955, despite the history of such suppression, the major determinant of family size had become the personal desire of the couple. Despite the continuing debates about the need for large families as a boost to the economy after World War II, the gradual transition to the role of the mother-as-worker, the general feeling about overpopulation in the Third World, and the increasing investment in contraceptive research and development eventually led to the development of an apparently safe intra-uterine device, and in the 1960s to an effective and reasonably safe anovulant pill. Reed argues that these major advances (often touted as *the* cause of a revolution in mores) were themselves responses to a changing cultural environment, particularly the modified role of the female. Her role changed from parent, helper, and companion in the home, to companion, parent, and wage earner; this trend, when joined with the feminists' movement urging the production of a female-controlled method of contraception, led to the 'pill', the key biomedical and pharmaceutical event which has since triggered more radical speculations which bear on the social mores.

H. Tristram Engelhardt reflects on the demise of the primacy of natural law. Natural law had prevailed before the development of highly effective contraception, which came to us in the way suggested by Professor Reed. Essentially, he says, while we are now allowed to view our sexual and aggressive impulses as 'natural' – since they are the result of evolutionary biological forces – we cannot accept all of them as moral. At the same time, the primacy of outside authority, whether divine or secular, no longer seems to us rational or even feasible.

Engelhardt argues that although it may still be problematic, sexuality with presumably effective contraception is less morally serious for us than sexuality without contraception. Therefore it is up to us to make new choices: (1) to fashion patterns of 'social and recreational sex', (2) to pattern our family lives in novel ways, (3) to choose work over child-rearing, and thus (4) inescapably to make many other novel choices as individuals. Sexuality is, he asserts, one of the central ways in which we endow our lives with content; the availability of freedom of choice, described by Judge Noonan, is thus only the first phase.

Section II opens with a paper by Thomas Halper, a political scientist, who seeks to set contemporary population attitudes in their historical context and to examine some of their more important implications. The 'population bomb' alarmists, he observes, are among the more recent of Malthus' innumerable progeny. But despite much hysterical talk, the rate of natural increase in the industrialized First World is minimal, and fears of overpopulation there now seem quite groundless.

Among the consequences of this development, Halper counts societies with higher mean ages, greater female participation in the workforce, and heightened concern on the part of traditionally dominant segments who may feel threatened by population growth among other groups. These societies may feature less anti-social behavior, a more dependable labor force, and more emancipated women. But they may also feature more strident generational and intergroup conflicts, a preoccupation with security at the expense of innovation, and child rearing practices of mixed results. Given these problems and its sharply decreasing share of the earth's population, can the First World maintain its primacy, politically, economically, and militarily? And if its influence shrinks, what will be the impact of this development internationally?

Halper then turns to the Malthusians, marshalling data to suggest that population growth, far from being the sure road to catastrophe, may be quite compatible with rising living standards. Discussing the concept of demographic transition, he also indicates that population growth may be self-limiting and that modernization and development may be a precondition for population control at least as much as population control may be a precondition for modernization and development. Then, stressing the advisability of caution in government efforts to regulate population growth, Halper emphasizes the inherent uncertainty of the future and humanity's capacity to shape its own destiny.

Jonathan Lieberson, a philosopher, addresses the difficult question of 'population ethics': Is it necessary or right in today's world for governments to seek to control the growth of population for their nations or for other nations? Lieberson asks, first, whether a consensus exists concerning the relationship of population growth to political instability or ecological disaster; he finds none. How to define the welfare of a nation with respect to this problem of population growth is, of course, the most intricate of problems – with or without actual consensus as to whether disaster lurks where population grows.

Searching for a method of approaching the problem, Lieberson stresses the point that moral theories may inevitably all be contextual – that is, they pertain to a given nation's specific situation. Thus, all such moral theories need to be scrutinized and considered as instruments, not as yielding totally formed plans or clear and comfortable sets of directives. They need to be employed when the routine or non-reflective response is no longer sufficient.

Lieberson then turns to the idea of governmental intervention and the rather limited circumstances under which a morally sound government decision to intervene might be reached and implemented. He does not preclude the need, within democratic review processes, for coercive action, but only contemplates them within those processes. He argues that although the preservation of basic human rights is often in question, these cannot be defined easily, since they are inextricably linked to their specific societal context – that context out of which conflicts of values have arisen. This, he argues, is not to deny such rights or succumb to moral relativism, but rather to recognize that the existence of a right does not make it universal and thus detached from consideration of all contextual factors.

Lieberson reviews a few actual instances of government action designed to reduce population in the 20th century; while these policies might seem unwarranted or extreme to American readers, he argues again that the values of those involved and the claims of the communities affected ought to be the principal factors influencing the decision to implement a program of incentives or restrictions, with preference given to 'softer', less coercive measures.

In an example – the case of politically organized peer pressure against increased births – Lieberson (without prejudging a large number of possible alternatives) insists upon employing specific democratic procedures: (1) the right on the part of those involved to be heard and, (2) having been heard, the right to be protected from serious and adverse consequences.

Lieberson is thus skeptical of many current approaches to the problem of population control, which typically emphasize protecting those rights assumed to be basic, without being proven to be basic. He is skeptical when any analysis disregards or neglects to consider seriously a specific political system or systems.

The China of today, for example, is attempting population control on a vast scale. The ethical questions raised by China's attempt are fascinating – politically, economically, and with respect to social justice —— as Janet W. Salaff, a sociologist, delineates them.

Salaff gives a detailed account of the great changes that took place in the cities and villages of China in the pre-revolutionary period, and their effect upon the traditional Chinese family, which had depended for its prosperity – indeed sometimes for its survival – on numerous and vigorous offspring. The radical political changes set in motion by the revolution marked a new social and cultural order, but the Chinese continue to depend almost entirely upon the traditional patrilocal family and the labor of all its members. In the first years of the new government, in fact, high fertility was supported as a matter of social justice; it was not until 1970 that numerous birth control campaigns began. Salaff then examines the urban changes which began to support the possibility of smaller families, and the large population growth which in the 1970s began to outstrip increases in food production. Here, the leadership believed, was *the* threat to social stability which justified truly extensive interventions.

According to Salaff, prior financial support provided to larger families was withdrawn, and a whole range of other opportunities for the children (e.g., to change jobs or be admitted to school) and for the parents (e.g., old age support) were also denied. Then even harsher sanctions were imposed on families with three children. Thus the family which insisted upon two or more children was subject to harsh economic sanctions and was deprived of certain opportunities for schooling or for job mobility. Parents with a third child might actually be docked work points (the numerical basis of wage income) or receive even further economic penalties.

In the face of such punishment, what could induce a family to contravene the perceived public good? How could such an important policy possibly fail, if in the future it should be found that excess population persists? These questions are raised whether or not the one-child policy has resulted in a rise in female infanticide. While the campaigns have apparently resulted in increased access to contraception (other than abortion), their intensity has resulted in this major political issue. Will so much change under conditions of uncertainty result in unbearable stress on the political fabric? Currently, there is enormous social pressure on all citizens to comply with this policy; is too much uniformity, too much change in this area politically dangerous?

Salaff examines the divergent situation in the cities, where the preconditions for material prosperity are quite different and where the family is much less important. New technology bearing on human reproduction and contraception (such as the radically new techniques of gene splicing, in-vitro fertilization and embryo transfer, genetic screening, and artificial insemination, as well as new contraceptive techniques) has brought us vast new responsibilities as the number and quality of choices increase.

Hans-Martin Sass, a philosopher, argues that changing technological realities always mean or *should mean* a greater emphasis upon personal responsibility. In a culture such as ours, which already reflects value pluralism, Sass holds,we have cultivated and must now further address our moral and legal responsibilities. Assuming that choices must be made, who shall grant rights or take up the responsibilities for making choices, Sass asks? Interventions may run from extremely indirect recommendation to legal directives. However, the starting point for discussion must be the responsible individual in an open society, if one wishes to argue from a Lockean standpoint.

The responsible individual is the only moral platform from which to discuss and argue among choices; it should be attempted, Sass argues, on the basis of the record of the enormous benefits made available to us through the achievements of modern science and technology.

Sass holds, optimistically, that a very high or near-perfect degree of control over fertility is possible; moreover, we have a responsibility to provide the next generation with the 'best possible' number of and best educated persons in that generation – a responsibility quite awesome for any society to accept. He assumes (unlike Lieberson) that it is not only possible to ascertain what population policy fits a generation's idea of optimum life and social conditions, but that we can and should actually determine how many people are best.

Sass recognizes that in an open society population policies may conflict with religious teachings, but he makes the point that there may be limits to the burdens which a society is prepared to bear due to the extensive power of particular religious groups. He apparently views accommodation by or persuasion through the group as quite possible. Given the complex and somewhat inconsistent history of 'contraceptive theology' which is reflected in the doctrines of the Roman Catholic Church, Sass sees room for accommodation, noting evidence of an ever growing separation between lay behavior and formal papal teaching. For Sass, religious teaching need not present an insuperable barrier to confronting ethical issues in a pluralistic society.

Sass concludes that entirely new responses to the phenomena of procreation, contraception, parenthood, and population need to be sought out. We can even contemplate new areas of socialization, if we conclude that the traditional family is inadequate or incomplete in the context of the necessary societal changes that we must face. Or, one may argue for perpetuation of the traditional family as a bulwark in times of drastic change. Sass argues (in the important area of population policy) for the responsible consideration of alternatives which least thwart individual choice. He judges as ethical the policy of compulsory sterilization which was put into effect in China, for under China's circumstances uncontrolled fertility was a severe and overwhelming hardship on and injustice to the community. Unflinchingly, he asserts that citizens in an open society must contemplate their responsibilities – to responsibly use new technologies – and thus 'rights' in this context, he says, are not necessarily fundamental, but should only follow or accompany our responsibilities to ourselves, others, and future generations.

Section III, "Social Responsibility and Public Policy", opens with a legal perspective. The development of doctrine and legal analysis depend upon the elucidation of 'rights', according to the attorney, Nancy N. Dubler, whether these rights are clearly defined or not. In the history of legal issues related to reproduction and fornication, the development in this century of specific rights to practice certain behaviors has been rapid, frequently discussed under the rubric of the 'right to privacy' or the 'right to informed consent' (when, for example, refusing medical treatment such as sterilization).

The right to use contraception, in our century, was one of the rights guaranteed under the 'right to privacy', and it was guaranteed first as a basic and fundamental right of married persons, and then of unmarried persons. Once this occurred, Dubler argues, it is not surprising that this 'right' soon extended to the virtually unrestricted right of a pregnant woman to elect abortion during the early stages of pregnancy but prior to fetal viability.

The right to reject medical assistance has a long history, and more recently this 'right' (called the 'right to informed consent') has been undergirded by the same broad concept of privacy, or the right to be left alone. This right has been crucial to the prevention of coercive sterilization which in the past had been visited upon women in the hands of misguided or even unethical medical authorities. The concept of 'privacy' in the law may not be sufficiently well-defined to differentiate, in some cases, the rights of the severely handicapped person to appropriate medical treatment, Dubler argues; however, on the edge of the area of sexual ethics and expression, the development of privacy rights raises fascinating and urgent questions: (1) In those states in which prohibitions against sodomy have been dropped or rendered unenforceable, is the privacy right of homosexuals now equal to that of heterosexuals? (2) If private, consenting conduct is protected in a fundamental way, then what state interest (e.g., the public's health interest in preventing the spread of the AIDS virus or herpes) is so overriding as to prohibit newly-protected behaviors? The prohibition of private sexual behavior on public health grounds has never seemed feasible or desirable in the U.S. What will be the next stage of legal development here? Dubler also asks whether the protection of privacy will extend to providing opportunities for sexual expression to those otherwise deprived of them – the incarcerated criminal or the institutionalized mental patient. These are some of the questions that must be addressed when, in the future, we employ and appeal to the notion of a 'right to privacy'.

Constance A. Nathanson, a professor of sociology, examines the relationship between our current idea of the appropriate public response to the sexually-active minor, and the message which soon reaches the client population, as delivered by nurses who are charged with providing actual services to them.

At least, according to their professed purposes, it is not the duty of nurses in public health clinics (who provide information to vast numbers of teenagers concerning contraception) to deliver lectures on moral behavior to teenagers. Nevertheless, as it happens, many of these nurses are married and have raised children. While many of them disapprove of the sexual activity of their clients, it is not, as they see it, appropriate for them to display disapproval by withholding services or delivering lectures – they are not *in loco parentis* in their clinical role.

Certainly, in the broader population there is significant ambivalence and even disapproval of the sexual activity in which these teenagers – whose median age is 16 – are engaged. Nathanson argues that since the medical profession has co-opted this conflict-laden area of personal behavior, religious morality has been replaced by medical morality. The nurses may well end by delivering a message of responsibility, autonomy, and good behavior, but only as it relates to the clinics' procedures: medical exams, returning regularly for 'pill'-prescription refills, or being conscientious about taking the 'pill'. A 'bad' patient may engage in unmarried sex, but must definitely take her pills regularly, without fail, or face the consequences. Failure is the 'fault' of the client. Nathanson points out that the lack of follow-up and a lack of empathic understanding of the problems of following a contraceptive regimen (with certain side-effects which may deter consistent use), may possibly result in a higher failed compliance rate for the client population. In short, the methods and message delivered to the clients may not be the most effective ones for them. Thus, Nathanson demonstrates that the sexual revolution, as it pertains to the younger and more vulnerable participants, has in fact produced a conflict of moral values, which still leaves this group in a disadvantaged position.

William B. Bondeson, a philosopher, comments on the implications of some of Nathanson's findings concerning the role of public health providers of contraceptive information. He notes that Dubler, among others, supports the lack of consensus concerning acceptable sexual behavior, and supports our regard for personhood based upon the moral and legal principles of autonomy and the right to privacy. These permit us to restrict the sexual expression of others *only* in the presence of demonstrable harm, either to themselves or to others.

The situation described by Nathanson suggests, to Bondeson, some distinct areas in which the concept of harm might be investigated, e.g., the weakening of the traditional family as the result of seeking and eventually obtaining contraceptive information. For Bondeson such concerns deserve serious attention. Furthermore, although the role of the medical provider may be described as educational, the question emerges whether the medical educator can sufficiently control his personal ambivalence about striving to increase the autonomy of the pupil (client). Perhaps no educator should restrain the initial impulse to impart values or norms, while providing information which may be valuable to the pupil's (client's) personal autonomy and freedom, especially if the biases of the teacher may in fact serve to undermine or defeat the original educational purpose. This is, of course, the question previously raised by Nathanson. Moreover, should the educator (nurse) take the moral responsibility for the consequences, if the educational practice should fail and the client become pregnant unwillingly? This is a dilemma for any educator.

Meredith W. Michaels, a philosopher, introduces Section IV by arguing that despite technological inventiveness which is effective and can make a crucial difference to a woman, women in general are not truly free either to have or not have children, simply because of the available technology. The key determinants of this kind of decision have always been general population need, mortality rate of infants and mothers and, most particularly, beliefs about reproduction and the good of society which result from particular rates of reproduction.

Michaels holds that women are permitted control over their own reproduction today only because they are needed for other work as new wage earners. Our economic situation thus requires that we accommodate their need to be free of child-bearing; thus their freedom is purely a conditional one. In a world of commerce such as ours, Michaels argues, certain energies must be concentrated on commercial activity, and on little else. Motherhood means a lengthy hiatus from the workplace in an activity which for a woman, because of her upbringing to be a mother, is especially immersing and distracts her from her previous role as worker. Moreover, continuously to be involved in the workplace requires her to continuously adapt, or appear to adapt, to a role for which she was not naturally raised. In this context, the 'choice' to become a parent cannot be said to be freely chosen; the context is too complex, and is thus the critical inhibiting factor which yields the illusory freedom of the adult woman of today.

Robert C. Solomon, a philosopher, asks the question whether contemporary technology actually 'frees' our sexual behavior. He answers that in fact our conceptions of sex have not been radically altered due to the technology of contraception.

First, Solomon points out, sexual behavior remains at the heart of our idea of morality. Our attitudes about sex still determine the acceptability of contraception, at least as much as the converse. The human purposes of sex include an enormous range of symbolic and practical concerns; the idea of a simple 'sexual instinct' was in fact a fabricated 19th-century concept. In actuality, sex is not a distinct activity or a pure, that is, isolated impulse. Moreover, it is not true historically that in the absence of effective contraception attitudes toward sex were timid and fearful. The correlation, historically, between reliable contraception and fulfilling sexual activity is 'most unclear'. The most important determinants have been social attitudes toward population and the practicality of having children. The social politics of classes and inheritance rights tended to predominate, and 'sex' was and is a political concept. Heterosexual intercourse is the convergence of many paradigms: the reproductive paradigm, the pleasure paradigm (that prevailed in the 1960s), the metaphysical paradigm (that of romantic love) and the intersubjective paradigm (where sex is a battle between domination and personal freedom).

Solomon argues that while Freud was the true architect of our ideas about sex – that pleasure by itself is not and has not been the true end of sexuality – this is by far too simple an explanation. He offers his set of paradigms as a way of canvassing the purposes of this complex human activity.

Stuart F. Spicker, a philosopher, in a closing commentary on

Michaels' and Solomon's essays, holds that they share a joint message: new contraceptive means are not the woman's means of changing her destiny, nor have these means radically changed our ideas about human sexuality.

As to Michaels' conclusion – that women are still bound by the social and economic restraints of the day and that their control over their own sexuality is simply conditional – Spicker parses the argument a bit finer and insists that even if the female role has not been revolutionized by recent developments (including sophisticated modes of contraception), still, control over one's own sexual life (during those years prior to the decision to have children) is now attainable, completely and without restriction for many if not most women. Surely this is an important change that demands our attention. As to Solomon's argument – that existing attitudes determine the degree of interest in contraception – Spicker points out that the advanced state of medicine, including ever new forms of contraception, can help us avoid the undesirable consequences of sexual activity more than at any time in history, and this possibility has had a significant effect upon our attitudes about engaging or refusing to participate in such activity. Perhaps, in the end, it is the magnitude and extreme suddenness of the transition to the new contraceptive ethos that has prevented us from imagining the various possibilities which may lie before us: indeed, we may soon have to accommodate ourselves to a fundamental and radically novel 'cosmology of sexuality'.

In any event, since it is clear to almost everyone that sex on satin surpasses sex on paper by such an order of magnitude that it is amazing that anyone would write on the subject at all, in retrospect we may come to appreciate the efforts of all the contributors to this volume who have addressed the plethora of concepts germane to the new contraceptive ethos and the issues of rights and responsibilities this movement has engendered.

March, 1987   STUART F. SPICKER

SECTION I

THE CONTRACEPTIVE ETHOS AND THE NEW BIOLOGY

THE HISTORY OF CONTRACEPTION: SEVEN CHOICES

Let me begin with some personal history. When I was a boy growing up in Massachusetts, the subject of today's lecture first intruded on my consciousness when, amidst the exuberant foliage of a New England fall, billboard advertisements appeared announcing that "Birth Control is Against God's Law" and urging, "Vote No On Proposition Six". An election was in progress, a referendum was being held on the Commonwealth's law banning the sale of contraceptives, and I began to wonder why birth control was against God's law. The argument which then appealed to me – I do not say it does so now – was that it was not against God's law to cut our fingernails; why should it be to curtail our other natural products?

Much later, at the University of Notre Dame, a colleague urged me to write the history of Catholic thought on this topic. I had already written a history of Catholic doctrine on usury and its development. He suggested I would find parallels. I doubted it. To begin with, I did not believe that the history of contraception could go back beyond the time when reliable contraceptives were discovered. I imagined the history of contraception to be a self-cancelling phrase like 'Swiss Navy'. But I thought I would take a look.

Since that date, twenty years ago, I have written a history of the Catholic teaching, a book which begins millennia before the birth of Christ. I have also analyzed the arguments pro and con the teaching, related the issues to demographic history, traced the new development in the encyclical *Humanae Vitae*, and charted the broader history of contraception in civilizations from Hindu India to Communist China. I do not propose to restate this work here, but to draw on it synthetically to present seven choices which have been made in the approach of human beings to contraception. As my two autobiographical stories may suggest, the history of contraception has depended as much on religious and philosophical evaluations as on the existence of technological means to accomplish a contraceptive end [10, 11, 12, 13].

Here are the seven choices:

3

Stuart F. Spicker, William B. Bondeson, and H. Tristram Engelhardt, Jr.
The Contraceptive Ethos, 3 14.
© 1987 by D. Reidel Publishing Company.

1. THE CHOICE TO TREAT THE SUBJECT SERIOUSLY

Contraception may readily be regarded as a trivial matter – my argumentative analogy with fingernail cutting suggests just how trivial. A civilization that appears to me to have treated it as morally trivial is Islam. The *Canon of Medicine* of the great eleventh century philosopher-physician ibn Sina is filled with accounts of potions, pessaries, and physical exercises to be used preventing conception. They are listed as remedies for the common cold might be listed in a physician's desk reference book today ([1], pp. 163, 277, 495). No moral note or caution is attached to their use. Nor have I found in any account of Islamic thought – certainly not in the Koran itself – any prescriptions of a moral kind governing their use. From the evidence I am familiar with, contraception in classical Islam was a non-moral subject, and – a corollary – not a serious subject.

In contrast stand the societies which have attached importance to the contraceptive act. Judaism is illustrative. Whatever modern exegesis or casuistry contends was the original sin of Onan in the Book of Genesis, the talmudists treated his spilling of seed in intercourse as a serious sin in itself [3, 8, 21]. As for the use of contraceptive drugs, these were debated by rabbinic Judaism and argued over on a case by case basis. There was no disposition to let the topic go or say that it didn't matter. Contraception had to be justified circumstantially. Discussion of the topic occurred within the context of belief in a duty to propagate the race until the Messiah came. With that duty understood as an obligation enjoined by God, the control of conception could not be regarded as wholly a private matter without social or religious implications [8, 18, 21]. Christianity inherited the basic Jewish concern and, for a long time, made the ban on contraception more absolute than had the talmudic casuists ([10], pp. 104–106).

It was possible, however, to take contraception more seriously than the Christians – to conceive of it not as a practice to be shunned, but as a duty to be observed. Such, in effect, was the position of the Manichees as reported by their opponents and as confirmed by their own documents. The central belief of this Persian religion, widespread in the fourth century Roman empire, was that there was a Father of Lights whose kingdom had been invaded by the King of Darkness, and the princes of darkness had defeated and devoured the princes of light; and after devouring the princes of light, the princes of darkness had copulated with the princesses of darkness; and from that union of devils there had issued man. Man is the child of darkness but contains within himself particles of light from the devoured princes of light. Creation is organized as a rescue of these particles, which seek their original home with the Father of Lights. The one great sin for man is to imitate the action of his devilish ancestors and procreate, for procreation perpetuates the imprisonment of the particles of light. Sexual intercourse is not banned, but procreative intercourse is. Contraception, practised by drug or by calculation of the fertile period, becomes a duty.

This religious belief which, in bold outline, may seem to us so crude and so incredible, was in its day sufficiently subtle and powerful to capture the minds of many intellectuals including for twelve years that of Augustine of Hippo. The Manichean world view, its sense of light struggling in conflict with a world of darkness, is not so different from several modern world views of human alienation – views which lead to a distaste for procreation if not to a prohibition of it. In the Manichean case, contraception or abortion was mandatory if sexual intercourse was to be enjoyed [5], ([10], pp. 106–112, 119–121).

When did contraception begin to be taken less seriously by Christians? The inference from demographic studies is that this change occurred at the time of the French Revolution. Nothing in the Reformation brought about a change, nothing in the Enlightenment in itself did so. But at the time of the Revolution, 20,000 Catholic parishes became vacant. Direct contact of Christian educators with the French populace largely ceased. The birth rate of France began to fall precipitously. It is a reasonable inference that both abortion and contraception began to be practised on a large scale by persons no longer instructed in Christian doctrine; and the practices were reinforced by the rationalists' insistence on the autonomy of man ([10], pp. 387–394). The demographer Alfred Sauvy calls this decline in the French birth rate at the height of Napoleon's victories the most significant fact in French history, and French nationalists as well as Catholics regretted it ([16], p. 13). At this point, however, for the first time in Western European history, contraception escaped religious control and became a matter of individual option, unburdened by serious moral objections. The modern battle over contraception was just beginning, but now a substantial portion of the population did not regard the matter as involving a law of God.

2. THE CHOICE NOT TO BE GOVERNED BY TECHNOLOGY

The ancient Egyptians had a formula employing crocodile dung intended to prevent conception, and it is a fair generalization that nearly
every tribe or people in nearly every age have had expedients intended to
work as contraceptives. The standing problem prior to modern time was
the lack of controlled experiments – the problem of ancient medicine
generally, so that the efficacy of many remedies remained unestab-
lished. There were also physical means of having intercourse without
insemination, and of course, as long as these were faithfully carried out,
sexual pleasure could be had without procreation. Finally, there was
information – usually wrong and counterproductive – as to the likely
period of fertility for a woman ([10], pp. 98–29, 120, 155–162).

If the morality of the use of contraception were to be decided only by
the availability of the means for accomplishing it, there was no reason at
any time to prohibit or limit the practice. Some effective techniques
existed. Other techniques may have worked at times, or worked sporad-
ically. "If it's there, use it", appears to be a peculiarly modern attitude;
but it was also the attitude of much of Greek and Roman medicine
about contraception, and the same attitude appears to be adopted in
Islam by ibn-Sina. In Greek and Roman society this attitude was
combated by a number of physicians committed to the philosophy of
Stoicism. For these latter physicians, considerations of nature were
prominent. As the eye is to see, they reasoned, so the genital organs are
to generate. It was unnatural to prevent the accomplishment of this
natural end. Yet this position did not necessarily impel them to an
absolute avoidance of contraception, but care and circumspection in
recommending it. They did not immediately conclude from the availability of the technology to its desirability ([10], 46–49).

In modern times, it is evident that both attitudes toward technology
have been present. "Things are in the saddle and ride mankind",
Emerson observes, and in general we see a willingness to use any
technology that is in existence. The use of the photocopy machine to
destroy the law of copyright is familiar to all professors. Yet there are
points at which we draw back from technology. The great unease about
the use of nuclear weapons is an example. Where contraception is
concerned, it would be fair to say that the invention of oral contraceptive drugs in the 1960's was a substantial factor in the spread of

contraceptive acceptance and became a reason for asking the Catholic Church to reconsider its universal prohibition. The papal commission on the subject was known in the Italian press as The Pill Commission. It is also fair to note that in the end the Pope refused to be influenced by the new means and by the distinctions which it afforded. Technological innovation may be decisive; it need not be; a choice always has to be made.

3. THE CHOICE TO BE GOVERNED BY THE END OR BY THE MEANS

When in 1793 Hung Liang Chi wrote his "Reign of Peace" and "Livelihood", he saw that in China overpopulation was linked to social misery. It was clearly a desirable goal to limit population growth. With this end in mind, Hung did not appear to have been concerned with the choice of means. Consequently, he gave no special emphasis to contraception as distinguished from cruder and more effective measures such as infanticide. In the same Chinese tradition, the nineteenth-century scholar, Wang Shih-to, recommended the postponement of marriage, the increase of nunneries for women, the forbidding of remarriage to widows, a tax on families with more than two children, the spread of drugs sterilizing women, and the killing of female babies at birth. These measures – obviously those of one we would classify today as a male chauvinist – seemed indifferent to him. They were all ways of reaching the desired end, the curbing of population growth ([4], pp. 271–274). When the means used were not considered significant, there appeared to be small reason to choose contraception as a favored technique.

Similarly, today, when in the minds of many persons any moral distinction has disappeared between abortion, contraception, and sterilization, there does not seem to exist for them any moral reason for emphasizing contraception. Health reasons may still make the latter preferable. But in popular understanding the difference between a back-up and a first-line remedy has become attenuated, especially since contraception requires foresight and advance planning, while abortion deals with the problem when it arises. In this society, modern America's, it is not surprising that there has been an increase in the number of abortions even as the availability of contraception has increased. The same correlation between rising abortion rates and acceptance of contraception has been found to exist in modern Japan ([9], p. 1252).

4. THE CHOICE OF QUALITY OR QUANTITY

There have been societies, or better said, governments for which the more, the merrier, has been the message. France after the Franco-Prussian war, Italy under Mussolini, Germany under Hitler, the Soviet Union under Stalin and his successors have actively propagandized to increase the population of the nation. The quality of the human life engendered has not been a concern. Contraception has been de-emphasized, discouraged, or, as in France after World War I, made, in various ways, illegal ([10], pp. 410–411).

Analogous rivalries between races (blacks and whites), between ethnic groups (Walloons and Flemings), between religions (Catholic and Protestant in Canada), between villages (contemporary India) have led one or both rivals to turn against contraception in an effort to beat the rival by creating superior numbers ([10], p. 353; [6], pp. 16–33). Wherever there is a perceived connection between power and popula-tion, and a perceived threat from a hostile group, the choice for quantity must operate to make contraception unattractive.

Another pressure for quantity has been religious —— in Hinduism, for instance, orthodoxy holds that a male descendant must be the person to perform the rites necessary to save one after death. When the doctrine is taken seriously, there is a desire to have a child, to have a male child, and to be safe by having more than one child. In contempor-ary India, Hinduism is one force leading Indians to question the value of contraception ([6], pp. 16–33).

The mainline Christian position on quantity has been different. Fa-voring virginity, celibacy, and maintenance of widowhood, early Christianity placed no premium on population increase. "The world is full" was a notion accepted by Gnostics and Christians alike. Apart from celebrating virginity, celibacy, and widowhood, Christianity taught that fornication was evil. The standard reason why it was evil, as developed by medieval scholasticism, was that it risked engendering a child deprived of paternal education. No the more the merrier in this view; rather, an insistence on the quality of the newborn's life. Finally and most centrally, Christian doctrine, from Clement of Alexandria on, held that the main purpose of Christian marriage was the procreation of offspring to be educated as Christian. In the classic phrase *bonum prolis* (the good or value of offspring), procreation *and* education of children were inseparably joined. The union of these two ends meant that procreation as such was incomplete, and numbers as an end in themselves unjustified ([11], pp. 465–470).

5. THE CHOICE OF MEANING FOR NATURE

Contraception is *contra naturam*, against nature, said the Stoics and the Christian Fathers and Thomas Aquinas. The charge is formidable, but what did they mean by "against nature"? Nature, the critic objects, provides mankind with a variety of diseases: it is human wit which overcomes the natural tendency of the body to degenerate and die. "If God meant us to fly, He would have given us wings" – nature in the sense of our original physical endowment is anti-scientific and anti-progressive. Man, living as naturally as possible, is a 'poor, forked creature'. It is clear that Christian tradition, so hospitable in fact to invention, has not meant by nature the unimproved condition of man ([12], pp. 234–235).

Does nature mean what animals do? Ludicrously, elephants have been cited by certain Christian writers as examples of chastity. On the other hand, doglike has been used as a pejorative for antiprocreative coitus. In fact, the animals have not been treated as normative, but as illustrative. Their sexual behavior has been used to provide images, not to ground an argument ([10], pp. 75, 77, 136, 163, 240–241, 248).

Is natural what occurs most often, so that the statistically probable is what is natural? There is an implicit acceptance of this view in the Kinsey report on human sexuality where the frequency of coitus by the respondents seems to function as a validation of certain kinds of sexual conduct. In this sense contraception is natural in our society. Yet nature in this sense of the ordinary or usual or probable is not what the authors of the Christian tradition or their Stoic predecessors had in mind. What is natural for them is what is in accordance with purpose. The unnatural is what is contra-purpose ([10], pp. 225–233).

"Whose purpose, and who determines it?" you may ask. On those questions, the traditional authors appear naive. Purpose appears to be equated with the biological function of an organ: as the eye is to see, etc. Who is to say? Apparently the rational philosopher or theologian is to say, after reflection on the uses of the organ.

This biological purpose view of nature is, however, accompanied in the great scholastic writers of the thirteenth century with a recognition that man's specific nature as human is rational. For man to act naturally is to act rationally. "Follow nature" is equivalent to the command, "Be rational". Implicitly, the purposes of the whole person, not the isolated organ, are the measure of the rational ([10], p. 235).

Such incipient rationalism, potentially so subversive of a merely physical understanding of nature, did not gain full recognition in the Catholic tradition until the Second Vatican Council. Then the Council in the pastoral constitution, *Gaudium et spes* taught that the criteria of judgment in matters of contraception came from "the nature of the person and his acts". A balance was attempted between the acts themselves and the person as a whole. What was natural was to be determined by looking at both [17].

It is on the basis of the Council's choice of this balanced meaning for nature that Pope Paul VI in 1968 was able to make a substantial advance in Catholic doctrine in *Humanae vitae*. According to this encyclical, the basic objection to contraception is "the indissoluble bond between the significance of unity and the significance of procreation" [14]. The basis of the Church's position, according to this reformulation, is not animal conduct or biological purpose, but the symbolic meaning of the connection between intercourse expressing love and procreation. In reference to the central symbolic significance of the procreative-unitive act, Paul VI said, "We think that the human beings of our age are most suited to see that this doctrine is consonant with human reason" [14]. What is natural is here treated as centered on the human person, as what is significant to human intelligence, as what is rational.

This restatement, this reformulation of the basis for objecting to contraception, has permitted commentators faithful to the encyclical to distinguish situations where contraception (a term not employed in *Humanae vitae*) violates the symbolic unity and cases where it does not. In the words of a distinguished French Jesuit, Father Gustave Martelet, explaining the encyclical which he helped prepare, "It is therefore necessary, at all costs, to distinguish between contraception and contraception" ([7], p. 1047). Concretely, contraception has been argued to be acceptable within the terms of the encyclical when it is practised in these situations: First, where there is no love being expressed in the coital act. Rape is the prime case here. The same reasoning would seem to apply in prostitution, casual fornication, and even in marriage where one spouse is forcing the other to intercourse against the other's will or when, say, in a drunken condition ([12], pp. 24–26). Second, when according to the normal rhythms of human fertility, the act should be non-procreative, for in such circumstances there is no necessary unity of the expression of love and fertility. In these cases, nature in the sense of statistical probability is introduced to determine what is normal. The norm appears to be four days of fertility per menstrual cycle. The employment of contraceptive means to assure that fertility is absent beyond the four days, is, it has been argued, consonant with the reasoning of the encyclical and the respect it accords both to the human person and the acts of the person. The underlying biological rhythm of fertility and sterility is accorded a normative value. It is left to the human person, recognizing this rhythm, to assure its certainty by contraceptive means ([12], pp. 24–26).

6. THE CHOICE OF PERSONS WHO ARE PERSONS

Who counts as a person? —— a fundamental question in any consideration of contraception. Are prisoners, slaves, blacks, women? Different societies have given different answers. The slave, a non-person in Roman law, is encouraged to practice contraception if what is wanted is availability for the master's sexual pleasure, or is discouraged from practising contraception if what is wanted is saleable progeny. The locus of the contraception decision is moved from the slave to the owner ([11], pp. 469–470).

Less brutally but not much less effectively, a given race – say blacks – may be discouraged from procreating by economic pressures, or may be treated as of such little account that procreation becomes a principal means of asserting their humanity. Women, as in many polygamous societies, may have such little personal dignity accorded them that it becomes essential to establish their claim upon their husband by motherhood. Such, in a famous biblical case, is the situation of Anna, the mother of Samuel [15].

Personhood becomes important in another way when means of controlling population are considered. If infants are not persons, there is no very strong sentiment against killing them – see nineteenth-century China ([14], pp. 58–61). If unborn children are not persons, there is no law against aborting them even at seven or more months. The absence of personhood for these classes means that contraception will not be seen as a uniquely desirable way of controlling the number of one's offspring.

Personhood has a third aspect. If persons are taken as, in some sense,

absolutes – as the ends for whose sake government exists, the decision
to procreate may be recognized as peculiarly personal, a right not to be
infringed by Church or State. In the United States, one class of human
beings has been denied this personal freedom – those classified as
mentally defective like Carrie Bell, whose forced sterilization by the
Commonwealth of Virginia was held by Justice Holmes to be constitutional [2]. Later Supreme Court decisions, however, have affirmed the
right to procreate to be private and beyond governmental interference.
In the light of such decisions – *Skinner v. Oklahoma*; *Griswold v.
Connecticut*; *Eisenstadt v. Baird* – it is doubtful that an American
government could make contraception mandatory [19].

A comparable position was taken by the Second Vatican Council. The
judgment as to the number of children they will have is a judgment, the
Council taught, which "ultimately the spouses themselves must make
before God" [17]. As Cardinal Wojtyla, later John Paul II, has said,
expounding the Council on marriage, "It is to the human person that
basic responsibility refers" [20]. Neither religion nor race nor ethnic
block nor tribal group has a right to override the two persons united as a
couple. The decision to practice contraception, as it now stands in the
American tradition, and the decision as to the number of children, as it
now stands in the Christian tradition, are decisions no one else can make
except the man and woman together, for themselves.

7. THE CHOICE OF BALANCE

Any viable ethic is a balance, a mix of values. The greatest of mistakes
in ethical reasoning, perhaps, is to suppose that an ethic as a whole is
determined by logic. Logic has a part to play. There are cases in which
he who says A must say B. But a very large part of the time Value A is
checked by Value B. There is no logical rule which tells you when this
limitation of A by B must occur. It is clear that Value A cannot be
permitted to eat up and destroy all the other values from B to Z. That is
the way of the fanatic, the dictator, the madman. It is also clear that
values B, C, and D need recognition, too. Balance is necessary. Experience, not logic, will tell you what balance is desirable.

The review of the six other choices which, historically, have effected
the acceptance of contraception has indicated some of the balances that
have been struck. This last choice is a reminder that every choice
affecting contraception will be part of a larger balance of values.

Advocates of Zero Population Growth ardently set out their goal in the 1960's, not shrinking from the recommendation of coercive techniques. Yet even in their zeal they struck a balance: they did not, for example, recommend the execution of an appropriate number of persons of childbearing ages; at this extreme point, respect for personal life and liberty inhibited them. Christians of earlier ages insisted that marriage has a procreative purpose. Nonetheless, at no time did the Christian Church bar marriage to those known to be sterile or past the age of childbearing. Again, respect for personal liberty prevented a too logical application of doctrine and led to a balancing of values ([10], pp. 129, 289–292). A third example: the right recognized in the person to make the basic decision to have or not have children – does it extend to the use of abortion or infanticide if a child has been conceived? Does it include the right to conceive a child in adultery, incest, fornication, polygamy or rape? Various values, apprehended differently by different persons, will be found in practice to limit a right so personal and so precious. Only a fanatic could say that the right, once recognized, eats up the rest.

Contraception, in summary, is an act, a practice, a lawful custom dependent on variable value judgments differently made in different epochs. As we try to understand its status today, we need not assume that the status will remain unchanged. The more it is taken as a serious matter, not dictated by technology, not the same as killing, not barred by a concept of biological determinism or a politico-social need for population, the more it is tied to nature understood as rational personhood, the more it is seen as an adjunct of love between persons in marriage, the more likely – I venture to predict – is its future assured.

University of California
School of Law
Berkeley

BIBLIOGRAPHY

1. Avicenna [ibn-Sinna]: 1582, *Canon medicinae*, trans. Gerard of Cremona, Venice, Italy, 2.2.
2. *Buck v. Bell* 274 U.S. 200 (1927).
3. *Genesis* 38:10.

4. Ho, P. T.: 1959, *Studies in the Population of China, 1368–1953*, Harvard University Press, Cambridge, Mass.
5. Mani: 1955, *The Treasure*, as quoted by Augustine, *De natura boni*, A. Moon (ed.), Washington, D.C., c. 46.
6. Mandlebaum, D.: 1974, *Human Fertility in India. Social Components and Policy Perspectives*, University of California Press, Berkeley, Calif.
7. Martelet, G.: 1968, 'Pour mieux comprendre l'encyclique "Humanae vitae"', *Nouvelle revue théologique* **90**, 1047.
8. *Niddah* 13a, 13b and 45a in the *Babylonian Talmud*: 1935–1952, trans. I. Epstein *et al.*, London, U.K.
9. Nizard, A.: 1970, 'Le Japon vingt ans après la loi eugénique', *Population* **25**.
10. Noonan, J. T.: 1965, *Contraception: A History of Its Treatment by the Catholic Theologians and Canonists*, Harvard University Press, Cambridge, Mass.
11. Noonan, J. T.: 1968, 'Intellectual and Demographic History', *Daedalus*, pp. 463–485.
12. Noonan, J. T.: 1980, 'Natural Law, the Teaching of the Church and the Regulation of Human Fecundity', *American Journal of Jurisprudence* **25**, 16–37.
13. Noonan, J. T.: 1965, '*Tokios* and *Atokion*: An Examination of Natural Law Reasoning Against Usury and Against Contraception', *Natural Law Forum* **10**, 215–235; Noonan, J. T.: 1979, 'Contraception', *Encyclopedia of Bioethics*, The Free Press, Macmillan, New York, N.Y., pp. 204–216.
14. Paul VI: 1968, *Humanae vitae*, *Acta apostolicae sedis* **60**, sec. 12.
15. 1 *Samuel* 1: 1–20.
16. Sauvy, A.: 1962, *La Prévention des naissances*, Paris, France.
17. Second Vatican Council: 1967, *Gaudium et spes*, sec. 50, 51, *Concilii Oecumenici Vaticani II Constitutiones, Decreta, Declarationes* (ed.) Florentio Romita, Rome, Italy.
18. *Shabbath* 110b in the *Babylonian Talmud*: 1935–1952, transl. I. Epstein *et al.*, London, U.K.
19. *Skinner v. Oklahoma* 315 U.S. 535 (1942); *Griswold v. Connecticut* 381 U.S. 479 (1965); *Eisenstadt v. Baird* 405 U.S. 438 (1972).
20. Wojtyla, K.: 1979, *Fruitful and Responsible Love*, Seabury Press, New York N.Y., p. 70.
21. *Yebamoth* 34b in the *Babylonian Talmud*: 1935–1952, transl. I. Epstein *et al.*, London, U.K.

HISTORY OF CONTRACEPTIVE PRACTICES

George Corner, the co-discoverer of the primary female sex hormone progesterone, began a history of reproductive biology with the first primitive agriculturalist who guessed that castrating male animals would improve their manageability and the quality of their meat ([10], p. iv). Corner's speculation that controlling the fertility of animals was a major step in human history, and an event related to the history of efforts to control the fertility of human beings, has been seconded recently by feminist scholars who have argued that the invention of animal husbandry some 10,000 years ago was intimately connected with new attitudes toward nature, women, children and sexuality (17).

As our ancestors turned from gathering to farming, and then to the animal husbandry, children were no longer loved as mysterious gifts from the gods and accepted for themselves alone. Rather, they became important sources of labor and a means of preserving family wealth; they were property. The relatively nonempathetic regard for and manipulation of women and children may have resulted from the dependence of farming people on the vagaries of nature, and the resulting vision of nature as an adversary or a force to be dominated and exploited for human benefit. Men learned to prune their herds ruthlessly, castrate or slaughter most male animals, while keeping as many females as possible for wool, milking and breeding. Lessons learned in managing animal fertility applied to human society. In turning from their original 'courteous' relationship with nature in which hunter and hunted were assumed to have mutual obligations and respect, men changed their relationship with all living things and discovered an advantage in controlling the reproduction of animals and women.

Since the invention of agriculture, no important culture has left the crucial business of reproduction to the choice of individuals, although one might argue that contemporary America is embarking on such an unprecedented experiment. In history, societies that survived necessarily developed hegemonic pronatal values. Social needs or goals are often at odds, however, with the interests and aspirations of individuals. Both

15

Stuart F. Spicker, William B. Bondeson, and H. Tristram Engelhardt, Jr.
The Contraceptive Ethos, 15–38.

anthropologists and historians have found widespread resistance, on the part of women and men, to the social imperative to produce children. Indeed, the Egyptian recipe for a contraceptive suppository of crocodile dung (1850 B.C.), described by Norman Himes in *Medical History of Contraception* [27], was but one of many such devices that Himes culled from the literature of ancient cultures; when these failed, women have resorted to abortion and infanticide on a startling scale [25, 29, 40, 34, 23, 26, 27, 49]. Throughout human history, the desire for children had to be taught and reinforced through social rewards and punishments, rather than being an innate unaltered human drive [20].

In historical context, contraception has been the most humane and efficient means used by individuals seeking to avoid or to limit the burdens of parenthood. Indeed, childbearing was onerous for the majority of women, as Edward Shorter reminds us in his recent survey of maternal mortality and morbidity in Europe before the twentieth century [49]. Given the ubiquity and logic of the human desire to control fertility, it might seem quite remarkable that social authorities ranging from popes, to lawyers, to physicians made so few distinctions of any practical importance between contraception, abortion, and even masturbation. The imperative to increase and to dominate was so powerful that it had to be 'overdetermined' by a powerful array of sanctions against any behavior that would deny state, faith, race, or tribe its rightful majority.

Contraception was still a controversial practice in the United States in the 1960s, when a series of judicial decisions and changes in government policy marked the conversion of a private vice into a public virtue. While the birth control pill was being developed in Massachusetts in the 1950s, it was illegal to give contraceptive advice in that Commonwealth. In 1965 the Supreme Court declared unconstitutional a Connecticut law, passed in the 1870s, that prohibited contraceptive practice by anyone, married or single, adolescent or adult. There was no formally recognized place for contraception in federal social welfare policy before 1967, when Congress amended the Social Security Acts to include budgets for family planning in domestic maternal health programs and removed contraceptives from the list of items that could not be purchased with foreign aid funds. In 1970 Congress finally got around to removing contraceptives from the list of obscenities banned by the federal Comstock laws. In 1972 the Supreme Court established in

Eisenstadt v. *Baird* that the unmarried should have the same access to contraceptives as the married ([44], pp. 376–379).

It is no fluke that the legalization of 'non-therapeutic' abortion followed in 1973, because our culture had never made a very clear practical distinction between contraception and abortion; both were banned for 'reasons of state' that only began to lessen after World War II. This can be seen in the course of describing contraceptive practices in the United States over the last two hundred years, and the cultural circumstances that have determined both public and private attitudes toward contraception.

While efforts to separate sex from procreation are ancient and widespread, there were no social movements to justify or promote contraception before the nineteenth century. Individuals pursued their self interests through such practices as coitus interruptus, periodic abstinence, or by placing a sponge or rag in the vagina to create a barrier between sperm and uterus; but they did so in flagrant violation of official standards of sexual conduct. Beginning in the 1820s in England and the 1830s in the United States, however, a small number of free thinkers argued that family limitation would help the poor by limiting the labor supply, or that it would strengthen the family by easing the burdens of overtaxed parents ([45], pp. 6–7).

In the United States, marriage manual writers representing all ideological persuasions soon joined the public debate begun by a few iconoclasts. The family was undergoing rapid change as home and work place were separated, new white collar classes emerged, and the quest for economic opportunity led increasing numbers of young adults away from their families or 'communities of origin'. The new marriage manuals found a market among those who were no longer willing or able to depend on kin for personal advice, and who were attempting to cope with the contradictory demands of a new kind of family ([45], pp. 19–33).

Whereas men once married to gain a working junior partner in the family business, home and workplace began to separate with the rise of the factory and economic development. Increasingly, marriage was understood less as an economic alliance between kinship groups and more as a fulfillment of passion between two individuals. The expected result of heterosexual cohabitation inspired by sexual excitement (romantic love) might be ten to fifteen children, but that number of dependents represented an intolerable burden on the socially ambitious in an economy in which children were no longer economic assets and required large investments in the forms of Christian nurture and lengthy educations.

Nineteenth-century Americans responded to the new social environment of industrial capitalism and the companionate family ideal by dramatically lowering their fertility. Whereas the average native-born white woman bore seven or eight children in the late eighteenth century, by the middle of the nineteenth century she was the mother of five, by the early twentieth century the mother of three, and by the Great Depression she was no longer replacing herself. One of the remarkable features of the American demographic transition is that there were no large declines in infant mortality before the end of the nineteenth century. Several generations of American women had fewer children than their mothers, despite a murderous infant mortality, and social leaders wailed that they were shirking from their patriotic duty, committing 'race suicide' and sinning against Nature [45, 53].

The precise role of contraceptive practice in the American fertility decline is not clear because both instrumentally-induced abortion and sexual self-restraint came into vogue among the Victorians [40, 38], ([45], pp. 19–45). It is difficult to separate sexual repression or what nineteenth-century Americans more properly called self-control, from contraceptive practice, and unsuccessful contraceptors were probably willing to resort to induced abortion. What is clear is that nineteenth-century knowledge of the process of conception and technology were adequate to support the development of birth control methods that were effective enough to account for the American fertility decline ([45], pp. 3–18). Descriptions of rubber condoms, spermicidal douches, 'safe periods' that were indeed safe, and 'womb veils' or contraceptive pessaries were in nineteenth century tracts that reached a mass audience. It could be argued that there were no fundamental advances in contraceptive technology from the middle of the nineteenth century until the marketing of the birth control pill in 1960. This lack of progress was not caused by a lack of possible contraceptive means, but was the result of widespread anxiety over what might happen if it became too easy to avoid the burdens of parenthood ([45], pp. 34–45).

The contrast between the technically possible and actual social practice is illustrated by the history of the spring-loaded vaginal diaphragm that, in 1984, still represents a wise contraceptive strategy. The mid-century development of modern rubber manufacturing provided a flexible substance that made cheap vaginal diaphragms and condoms possible. As early as 1842, the German physician W. P. J. Mensinga took the ordinary hard rubber ring used for correcting uterine displacements and covered it with sheet rubber to form a diaphragm across the cervix. This device was much inferior to the contraceptive diaphragm with which we are familiar, however, for reasons explained in an 1878 patent application for an improved device:

A pessary of hard rubber is very stiff and liable to be broken, is uncomfortable to the wearer, and cannot be readily fitted to any patient . . . it quickly collects sediment, and emits an unpleasant odor . . . ([5], p. 106).

In 1846 the British chemist Alexander Parkes helped to remedy the situation by patenting the 'cold cure' process in which rubber was vulcanized instantaneously by treatment in a solution of sulfur chloride in carbon bisulfide. Parkes's discovery was important in the development of rubber manufacturing because it made possible the mass manufacture of thin delicate articles such as surgeon's gloves. With the availability of thin vulcanized rubber, Mensinga and a series of American physicians rapidly improved on their hard-rubber pessaries by making thinner, flexible devices with coiled springs in the edges to keep them in place. As the 1878 patent applicant explained:

This improved pessary may be bent or folded in any way necessary to apply it, and it will then spring outward under the action of its spring. This vulcanized soft-rubber covering, free from smell gained in use, and soft, so as to act as a cushion, and not inflame or feel harsh or chafe the parts, is a matter of great importance ([5], p. 106).

Apparently, the first American description of an improved 'womb veil' appeared in the 1864 edition of *Medical Common Sense* by Edward Bliss Foote, an 1858 graduate of Pennsylvania Medical University and popular medical journalist ([6, 7]). Foote's rationalization for the 'womb veil' is important in the light of the long hiatus between the time when the spring-loaded vaginal diaphragm was described by physicians and the clinical testing and statistical evaluation of this device in the 1920s. Foote boosted his pessary because he thought that douching caused leucorrhoea, that coitus interruptus was injurious to mental health, and because he abhorred the practice of abortion, "now so prevalent among married people". Also, the vaginal diaphragm "places conception entirely under the control of the wife, to whom it naturally belongs; for it is for her to say at what time and under what circumstances she will become the mother and the moral, religious, and physical instructress of offspring" ([19], pp. 380, 335–337). That, however, was precisely where the leaders of American medicine and society did not want control of conception to rest.

By the middle of the nineteenth century a voluminous literature defined 'the population problem' that would be an ever-present consideration in discussion of birth control, feminism, and the family until after World War II. One of the discoveries of Francis A. Walker (director of the 1870 United States Census) and other pioneers in the gathering of social statistics was the phenomenon of differential fertility among ethnic groups and classes. Walker, a proud Yankee, was appalled while standing in a voting registration line because illiterate Irishmen were extended the same privilege. The social tensions associated with mass migration were especially frightening because of the declining fertility among the native-born, and Walker became both an exponent of 'Muscular Christianity' and of immigration restriction ([45], pp. 197–202).

Physicians were also alarmed by the low birth rate among their paying customers and the apparent dissatisfaction of young women with their 'natural' roles as wives and mothers. Since the family might have been weakened if sex was too easily separated from procreation, doctors believed it was their duty to carefully manage the dissemination of birth control information [46]. While many of the most popular marriage manuals that included how-to sections on contraception were written by physicians, the leaders of the profession were hostile toward any means of family limitation. They were responsible for the mid-nineteenth century criminalization of all abortion.

Prior to 1830, the law on abortion was generally permissive. This casual attitude reflected the fact that there were no means of determining whether a woman was pregnant or simply 'irregular' before the fetus began to move in the womb; those seeking abortions were usually unmarried women, generally viewed as victims of male lust. Between 1840 and 1870 apparent changes in the social status of women seeking relief from pregnancy alarmed many physicians and led them into successful campaigns to outlaw induced abortion at any stage of pregnancy. As historian James Mohr has demonstrated, doctors believed that many married Protestant women began to seek abortions, and they seemed "to have been deeply afraid of being betrayed by their own women" ([40], p. 168). They reacted with denunciations of feminists and successful lobbying campaigns in state legislatures. By 1880 induced abortion was illegal, many wise-women and irregular practitioners had been driven out of business, and physicians gained new stature as moral arbiters.

Twentieth-century exponents of contraception often legitimated their cause by painting a horrible picture of poor women drawn into the hands of quack butchers due to the lack of legal and safe means of fertility control, but in the last decades of the nineteenth century neither physicians nor feminists were particularly interested in distinguishing between contraception and abortion. The systematic suppression of contraceptive information paralleled the outlawing of abortion. While the new ideal of companionate marriage based on romantic love might in retrospect seem to require recognition of erotic bonding and non-procreative marital sex, most Victorians remained preoccupied with the need to sublimate eroticism to higher ends. When the Comstock Act, a strengthened national obscenity law, was passed in 1873, no distinctions were made among smut, abortifacients and contraceptives – all were equally obscene, and explicit discussions of contraceptives were omitted from post-1873 editions of many books in which the subject had originally been given space ([45], pp. 34–45).

The need and desire of individuals to control fertility remained, however, as witnessed by the continuing decline in birth rates and the inability of physicians to avoid the subject. In 1898, the Physicians Club of Chicago sponsored a symposium on 'sexual hygiene' in order to provide an opportunity for frank exchange of information among doctors interested in becoming better marriage counselors. One of the participants explained, "Outside the medical profession it is taken for granted that the doctor knows all about these things [sex]. But within our ranks we are aware that this is not true. The textbooks omit this department" ([14], Preface). The public increasingly turned to physicians instead of the clergy for sex advice, but some physicians were willing to admit, at least among themselves, that they had insufficient knowledge of the subject. An edited transcript of the symposium was published as a 'for doctors only' handbook, entitled *Sexual Hygiene* [14], in an effort to meet the need for information.

The editors of *Sexual Hygiene* believed that husbands bore a major share of the blame for the marital unhappiness that seemed to be reaching epidemic proportions. Too many of them were ignorant of, or ignored, the sexual needs of their wives. Husbands had to be taught that "the God-given relation is two-sided, and that without harmony and mutual enjoyment it becomes a mere masturbation to the body and mind of the one who alone is gratified" ([14], p. 95). It was thought that better marital sex would lower the divorce rate and keep both husbands and wives at home where they belonged.

One chapter of *Sexual Hygiene* was devoted to contraception. Contributors ignored the illegality of the subject and accepted birth control as a necessary means, in some cases, of reconciling the economic and personal interests of husbands and wives. They knew of numerous contraceptive methods, but birth control information was given with discretion. There were situations in which it was kept from patients. "We all know perfectly the difference between the dragged-out woman on the verge of consumption, the rachitic pelvis, and the society belle, who mistakenly thinks she does not want babies when every fiber of her being is crying out for this means of bringing her back to healthy thought."([14], p. 184).

This ambivalent attitude toward birth control was most strikingly revealed in a long discussion of contraceptive methods. The strong-willed tried "limiting intercourse to the period from the sixteenth day after menstruation to the twenty-fifth". Men practiced withdrawal or used condoms. The condom was very effective, "if the best are used, but we all know that rubber is a non-conductor of electricity, and this is a factor that, I think, should not be disregarded. They are not the easiest thing in the world to put on either" ([14], pp. 188–190).

While a highly effective and safe contraceptive was mocked because it interfered with male pleasure, female methods received indiscriminate endorsement. "The little sponge in a silk net with string attached is a familiar sight in drug stores. If this is moistened with some acid or anticeptic solution before use and rightly placed it is very safe and harmless". In addition to the sponge, would-be female contraceptors might choose either douching, "a vaginal suppository of cocoa butter and ten percent boric and tannic acids", or "the womb veil with eight grams of quinine mutate to an ounce of petrolatum". All seemed to work well. A final bit of advice was offered for the woman who wanted to avoid having children without good reason: "Get a divorce and vacate the position for some other woman, who is able and willing to fulfill all a wife's duties as well as to enjoy her privileges" ([14], pp. 185–187, 189–190).

Although these physicians knew of many female methods, they were not concerned with making distinctions among them or with the problems that women had in using them. Systematic clinical evaluation of contraceptives did not begin until the 1920s, when minor improvements in the vaginal diaphragm provided the most effective female method available until the marketing of the anovulant pill in 1960. Serious study of birth control methods might have begun in the mid-nineteenth century because both the necessary technology and knowledge of sexual anatomy were available, but doctors did not make any major efforts to improve contraceptive means.

The participants in the Physicians Club symposium were typical of their age, and of twentieth-century social elites as well, in their willingness to sacrifice the desires of individuals to the social imperative to reproduce, but the suppression of contraceptive information did not change the pattern of declining birth rates. In 1901 the populist sociologist E. A. Ross coined the term 'race suicide', and President Theodore Roosevelt declared that America's future as a world power was being undermined by the pursuit of the soft life exemplified by barren marriages. Between 1905 and 1909 more than 35 articles appeared in popular magazines discussing the infertility of native Americans. The inability of many young adults to cope with the demands of 'civilized morality' provided the first generation of American specialists in psychotherapy with many cases of neurosis. The widespread idea that traditional somatic explanations of mental illness were inadequate was paralleled by the discovery of adolescence as a 'problem' and the invitation of Sigmund Freud to visit Clark University, where he explained how the tension between eros and civilization could lead to madness [24, 45, 46].

One of the best contemporary explanations of the so-called 'crisis' in civilized morality' was provided by the University of Pennsylvania economist Simon Patten. In 1905 Patten announced the arrival of a new era of abundance with a series of lectures that were published under the title *The New Basis of Civilization* [42]. Patten argued that the Protestant values of hard work and dedicated abstinence had been an important resource in American economic development, but the success of Protestant asceticism in promoting capital accumulation had led to an economic revolution symbolized by the giant corporation and mass production. In the new world of mass consumption and economic bureaucracy, Americans needed to learn how to consume. The heroic entrepreneur whose iron 'character' was appropriate to a society of scarcity was being replaced by the organization man whose other-directed 'personality' was expressed in the arts of leisure and consumption ([52], pp. 212–226).

Patten's call for new sexual attitudes appropriate to an affluent society was not heeded by most social arbiters who continued to fret over 'race suicide' and the equally threatening phenomenon of 'clandestine prostitution', or the appearance in public of large numbers of unchaperoned women ([9], pp. 40–41). As the dynamic service sector of the economy drew ever-larger numbers of women into jobs outside of the home, relations between the sexes began to reflect a new social reality. Married companionship had seemed the best that the nineteenth-century economy could support for its young middle classes. Young men and women in the early twentieth century sought the pleasure of companionship before marriage in the world outside the home. The generous figure of the Gibson girl was replaced in the popular imagination by a creature with slim hips and short hair, who played tennis or swam, danced the fox trot, smoked cigarettes, and necked with men she might not marry. The 'new woman' was a comrade in arms with male friends against the sexually segregated adolescence and exaggerated sex roles of their parents ([45], pp. 54–63).

As youth heard the appeals of the newly prominent advertising industry to relax, consume and enjoy, the traditional values of austerity and sacrifice that supported nineteenth-century sexual ideals eroded. Among the predominantly upper-middle-class women interviewed by Alfred Kinsey in the 1940s, those born between 1900 and 1909 set a pattern of premarital sexual behavior that remained essentially unchanged until after World War II. These women made necking America's favorite pastime, and 36% of them engaged in premarital intercourse. Premarital coitus among men born between 1900 and 1909 did not increase, and coitus with prostitutes decreased by over 50%; the slack was taken up by friends, two-thirds of whom were fiancées ([31], pp. 267–269, 300, 330).

The new courting pattern – prolonged heavy petting, sometimes leading to coitus, and usually followed by marriage – did not signal the collapse of monogamy, marriage, or the family. Rather it reflected the emergence of a single standard of permissiveness with affection. As the sociologist Ira Reiss shrewdly observed, the new standard did not mean frivolous sexuality or acceptance of 'body-centered' coitus. Sex as self-centered pleasure was the standard of men who avoided coitus with their fiancées because they were 'good girls' and sought relief with prostitutes [47].

Young people simply expanded the limits of the nineteenth-century ideal of companionate marriage and 'person-centered' coitus developed by their parents. Petting provided an opportunity for the sexes to learn to know one another. It was a necessary prelude to mature sexual relationships and an appropriate form of sexual expression for adolescence, the prolonged period of social dependency necessary for the middle classes in an industrial society. Kinsey's study showed a correlation between heavy petting and the ability of women to achieve orgasm in marriage. Sexual compatibility in marriage, in turn, was associated with a low divorce rate ([31], pp. 358–359, 371–373).

Both the nineteenth-century ideal of companionate marriage and the twentieth-century standard of permissiveness with affection were relationships based on mutuality and justified by affection. In the twentieth-century version of ideal love between man and woman, sex and procreation could be separated, but sex was still justified by the investment of much psychological capital in a stable relationship. Permissiveness with affection rested even more narrowly on intimate and personal values than the companionate marriage, and thus was more dependent on sexual attraction and fulfillment.

In retrospect, the emergence around 1915 of a movement to legitimate and spread contraceptive practice might be viewed as a logical, if not inevitable, response to one source of tension in the sex lives of socially ambitious Americans. The essential cultural prerequisite for public acceptance of the separation of sex from procreation was secularization of society or the celebration of material well-being and pleasure exemplified by the growth of the advertising industry. Many Americans were not ready to believe, however, that affection alone justified sex. A great majority of the more than 24 million immigrants to the United States between 1880 and 1920 had conservative attitudes toward sexuality. Their presence gave a tremendous boost to nativist anxieties over the future composition of the American population. The foreign- and native-born united in suspicion of those who wanted to change contraception from a furtive and illegal private practice into a legal and socially accepted right. For nativist and immigrant, Protestant, Catholic, and Jew, the population problem was not too many people but a dearth of people of the 'right kind', although the definition of 'right kind' varied.

Margaret Sanger is the best known twentieth-century advocate of contraception. Her biography and public career illuminate both the sources of support for and opposition to birth control. The third daughter in a lower-middle class family of eleven, Sanger bitterly resented the relative poverty of her large family and blamed her free-thinking Irish father for the death of her mother at the age of 49, a martyr to the burden of bearing and raising children. When at the age of 30 Sanger found herself a tubercular mother of three and trapped in a marriage with a man who had much in common with her father, she rebelled by joining the labor movement. Drawing upon her own experience as a nurse and the counsel of such rebels as the anarchist Emma Goldman, Sanger eventually established herself as a radical spokesperson on issues concerning women. It was Sanger who developed the strategy of justifying contraception by publicizing the appalling number of working-class women who died from septic abortions ([45], pp. 67–88).

Sanger's primary animus as a social reformer was an intense resentment of the liabilities women suffered because of unwanted pregnancies, and her career can be understood as a consistent quest for female reproductive autonomy ([45], pp. 129–139). She was a feminist, always depended on the support of other women, and consistently tried to represent their interests in the male-dominated forums where she was forced to plead her cause. After being arrested in 1916 for operating a contraceptive advice center, Sanger began to change her tactics and gradually abandoned the posture of militant woman rebel. In response to a 1918 New York state court decision that upheld her conviction but found contraceptive advice by a physician legal, and influenced by society women who proved to be her most consistent sources of financial and moral support, Sanger cultivated a new image as a married mother lobbying among legislators and professional elites. In building a coalition for birth control, she learned that the ideal of reproductive autonomy for women was literally a joke among the great majority of American male influentials ([45], pp. 99–105), but some doctors, legislators, and philanthropists supported her cause on other grounds.

During the decade before World War I, a number of prominent physicians were led, through their experience in such specialized practices as gynecology and pediatrics, to question the legal and social taboos on birth control. While they tended to be liberals on 'the woman question', these medical reformers were not feminists. They had become convinced that unwanted or ill-timed pregnancies posed a greater danger to stable family life than open discussion of sexuality. The most important of these pro-birth control doctors was Robert Latou Dickinson, who established the National Committee on Maternal Health in 1923, to lobby for medical sex research. Over a 20 year period Dickinson's committee published a series of authoritative monographs that convinced reluctant colleagues to accept contraceptive advice and marriage counseling as essential medical services ([45], pp. 143–193).

Dickinson found gathering empirical evidence on sexual behavior to be much more difficult than he anticipated, but in 1923, Sanger established the first doctor-staffed birth control clinic in the United States and began the arduous task of collecting the case records that would demonstrate the effectiveness and safety of contraceptive practice. After some experimentation, Dr. Hannah Stone, the clinic's medical director, determined that the method of choice should be a spring-loaded vaginal diaphragm used with a spermicidal jelly, and, in 1928, with Dickinson's assistance, she published the first large-scale analysis of case records from Sanger's Clinical Research Bureau [50] and definitively disproved the irresponsible claims by Morris Fishbein, editor of the *Journal of the American Medical Association*, that contraceptive practice did not work and often led to cancer or insanity ([16], pp. 55–56, 218–220, 142–149).

By the early 1930s a coalition of feminist and medical reformers had established a nation-wide network of birth control clinics that served as teaching centers for interested doctors and as sources of data for Dickinson's *Control of Conception* [12] and other authoritative pro-contraception monographs. In 1936 a federal judge recognized the empirical case for birth control in ruling that the Comstock Act should not close the mail to contraceptive information and supplies intended for physicians. Building on this legal exemption, in 1937 Dickinson engineered an American Medical Association convention resolution that accepted contraception as a legitimate service to be provided by the physician "largely on the judgment and wishes of individual patients" ([45], pp. 186–190).

The sex histories gathered by Alfred Kinsey reveal that the birth control clinics and lobbying campaigns among physicians led to important changes in contraceptive practice among the middle classes. (Table I) Of Kinsey's married white female subjects born before 1899, only

TABLE I
Kinsey's survey

	–1899	1900–09	1910–19	1920–29
Sample = 2,328	323	560	867	578
Never practiced				
contraception	12% (40)	7% (37)	8% (65)	5% (31)
Diaphragm	24% (77)	42% (237)	53% (455)	57% (327)
Douche	24% (76)	15% (85)	8% (66)	6% (35)
Withdrawal	23% (72)	15% (85)	7% (61)	7% (41)
Condom	36% (116)	37% (206)	34% (296)	37% (215)

12% claimed never to have practiced contraception. The main result of the birth control movement at the behavioral level among Kinsey's subjects was not the initiation of contraceptive practice but the substitution of the vaginal diaphragm for douching and withdrawal. Of the women born before 1899, 24% reported 'much use' of the diaphragm, but 24% relied heavily on douching and 23% on withdrawal. Among the women in the next three cohorts, 'much use' of the diaphragm greatly increased, while douching and withdrawal lost their popularity. Although Sanger wanted to place contraception under the control of women, the increased availability of the diaphragm did not lessen the popularity of the condom. Thirty-six percent of Kinsey's female subjects born between 1920 and 1929 still relied heavily on it. The condom's persistence in comparison to douching and withdrawal probably reflected its high effectiveness. Also, condoms were more easily and cheaply obtained than diaphragms, since one did not have to go to a doctor to be fitted ([45], pp. 123–126).

Sanger and Dickinson hoped that better contraception would lead to fewer induced abortions, but women born between 1900 and 1909 reported more induced abortions (29% had at least one) than those born before 1899. This difference might reflect the possibility that the older women in Kinsey's sample were recruited more heavily from religious groups than from other voluntary associations. The rise in induced abortion could be interpreted, however, as a reflection of a greater unwillingness to maintain unwanted pregnancies among women during the 1920s and 1930s. Possibly they were learning that effective contraception was possible, and were therefore less passive in the face of contraceptive failure. Only 17% of those born between 1910 and 1919 reported induced abortions. This decline reflected the relative youth of these women, who were between the ages of 30 and 39 when they were interviewed, but they might also have been more effective contraceptors and thus would have experienced fewer unwanted pregnancies ([45], pp. 125–126).

Although birth control advocates were able to lower the cost of practicing contraception for women who were willing and able to seek help from a birth control clinic or the minority of private physicians who offered contraceptive services, most sexually active Americans continued to doctor themselves. Among the first 10,000 patients at Sanger's Birth Control Clinical Research Bureau, less than 55% continued to use the diaphragm regularly after a year ([33], pp. 176, 193–194, 196). Mary McCarthy, in *The Group* [36], her evocative portrait of Vassar women from the class of 1933, provided a fictional but realistic description of the diaphragm's inherent drawbacks. In a genital-shy culture, even a Vassar woman had problems managing the gadget:

Dottie did not mind the pelvic examination or the fitting. Her bad moment came when she was learning how to insert the pessary by herself. Though she was usually good with her hands and well co-ordinated, she felt suddenly unnerved by the scrutiny of the doctor and the nurse, so exploratory and impersonal, like the doctor's rubber glove. As she was trying to fold the pessary, the slippery thing, all covered with jelly, jumped out of her grasp and shot across the room and hit the sterilizer. Dottie could have died. But apparently this was nothing new to the doctor and the nurse ([36], pp. 72–73).

Dottie left her new contraceptive under a park bench without using it.

Whatever the limitations of the existing technology in the 1930s, 13 million fertile married couples in the United States faced the question of whether to create a new life. While social scientists and politicians blamed the Great Depression on the low birth rate, ordinary people struggled to manage their own affairs, and in 1937 spent $38 million on condoms and over $200 million on 'feminine hygiene' ([45], pp. 208–209, 239–246). According to the law, contraceptives could only be sold with a medical prescription. Thus, condoms were "for the prevention of disease" and tons of douche powder passed over the counter in the name of internal cleanliness, despite agreement among medical authorities that the genital tract was self-cleansing and douching might cause disease.

The clandestine nature of the contraceptive industry allowed manufacturers and retailers to charge exorbitant prices. A gross of condoms that cost the manufacturer $4.80 and the druggist $6 retailed for $24, a markup of 400%. Because testing condoms almost doubled the cost of manufacture, many defective articles were sold. Advertisements claiming a product was 'sure, safe, and dependable' for 'feminine hygiene' were interpreted by the public to mean 'sure, safe, and dependable' for contraception. The result was an enormous amount of money spent on useless, marginally effective, or harmful products. A *Ladies Home Journal* poll showed 79% of American women 'believe in birth control'. They also considered four children the ideal. The most important reason why the two-child family was the behavioral norm was 'family income'. Thus, in the midst of the Depression, the American desire to maintain a decent standard of living was used to cheat them out of millions of dollars.

The National Committee on Maternal Health (founded by Robert Dickinson in 1923) was principally responsible for publicizing the scandalous practices in the birth control business with the result that the Food and Drug Administration began to test condoms and to confiscate defective articles; the AMA's Council on Pharmacy and Chemistry began to issue reports that defined standards for contraceptive products and listed the commercial brands that met the standards. Efforts to control the feminine hygiene racket were less effective. Peddlers of useless and harmful powders were fined and forced to change their advertising in a series of Federal Trade Commission actions, but the lack of a clear means of establishing the purpose and effectiveness of a product made suppression of the trade difficult. Also, the man who financed and orchestrated the Committee on Maternal Health's campaign to regulate the birth control industry, Dr. Clarence J. Gamble, an heir to the Ivory Soap fortune, knew that douching did reduce fertility, and he opposed complete suppression of "lay advertising as it had value in bringing to the attention of the public that there was such a thing as Birth Control" ([45], p. 245).

In contrast to Margaret Sanger, whose mission as a birth controller was to liberate women from unwanted pregnancies, or the majority of pro-birth control physicians, who hoped to strengthen family life through better marital sex, Dr. Gamble's principal concern was differential fertility among classes and the high cost of social programs for the poor ([45], pp. 225–238). While Sanger and Dickinson saw the birth control clinic as a way of bringing a new sense of self to women, Gamble chafed over the high cost of medical attention for everyone. During the 1930s, he initiated a series of remarkable experiments in the mass delivery of contraceptives and achieved some surprising successes. In Logan County, West Virginia, for example, door-to-door distribution of free lactic-acid jelly between 1936 and 1939 led to a 40% decline in birth rates among the poor women who were willing to try the method ([2], pp. 42–51, 53–54, 132–133, 152). In Logan, as elsewhere, Gamble's efforts ran into problems of cost and the reluctance of public officials to devote scarce resources to contraception. The annual cost per patient for distribution of contraceptive jelly by a nurse was less than $6, but in 1938 West Virginia spent $1.25 on public health per rural family. Birth control services seemed an extravagance beyond the means of private philanthropy or government. Gamble initiated other programs, distributing condoms in North Carolina, experimenting with foam-powder-on-a-sponge in Florida, and paying missionary doctors to show Indian peasants how to make a cheap vaginal barrier by dipping a rag in brine solution, but he remained a quixotic outsider, only slightly less influential than Sanger and Dickinson, until the redefinition of 'the population problem' provided a powerful new rationale for experiments in population control and innovations in contraceptive technology.

During the 1950s the social and political climate changed in ways that strengthened the hand of birth control advocates. First, married women with children were drawn in ever larger numbers into paid work outside the home ([4], [15]). The great majority of American families could not attain the American dream of ever-increasing affluence with a single income. This underlying economic and behavioral reality was reflected in a 1955 national survey of representative married women. By the end of their fertile years, 'substantially all' married couples had tried to regulate conception if they were not subfecund. Half began contraceptive practice before the first pregnancy, an additional 32% before the second, 11% more before the third. Their reasons were overwhelmingly economic, although Catholics were more likely than Protestants to mention health as a rationale. The researchers concluded that, "The major determinant of family size in the United States is the number of children that couples want to have" ([21], pp. 62, 168, 257, 402). Even more important for the future of public policy on reproduction: "All classes of the American population are coming to share a common set of values about family size." More couples wanted five or more children than none at all, but most wanted between two and four and actually had two or three.

Despite the almost universal determination of married couples to limit their families, and their successful contraceptive practice, birth control remained a controversial political issue because of the opposition of the Roman Catholic hierarchy and the feeling on the part of most non-Catholics that higher birth rates were good for the economy. In June, 1958, the cover of *Life* magazine showed several dozen infants modeling expensive walkers, rockers, and other 'kiddie-care' paraphernalia under the headline, "Kids: Built-in Recession Cure", but in July a controversy broke out in Brooklyn that marked the point at which even the Catholic Church tacitly began accepting the consensus on family planning.

Dr. Louis M. Hellman (later first director of population affairs in the United States Department of Health, Education and Welfare during the Nixon administration), a gynecologist at King's County Hospital, a tax-supported municipal institution, decided to defy the *de facto* regulation against birth control services in public institutions. His well-chosen martyr was a diabetic Protestant, two of whose three children had been delivered by caesarian section. The city commissioner of hospitals honored the traditional understanding among Catholic, Protestant, and Jewish politicians by ordering Hellman not to fit his patient with a diaphragm, but during the ensuing controversy, skillfully orchestrated by the Planned Parenthood Federation of America, important divisions emerged in the Catholic community. *Commonweal*, the lay Catholic magazine, editorialized that: "Where consensus once existed, it no longer does . . . . . There are many sound and compelling reasons why Catholics should not strive for legislation which clashes with the beliefs of a large portion of society" [8]. Eventually, the New York City Board of Hospitals voted eight to two to lift the ban on contraception, and the emergence of John F. Kennedy as a serious contender for the 1960 Democratic presidential nomination provided both Catholic bishops and laity with powerful incentives for avoiding controversy over issues of Catholic power in shaping public policy ([35], pp. 22–24).

As Catholic opposition to contraception softened, 'the population problem' was being redefined in ways that undermined the traditional consensus on the benefits of population growth. After World War II, influential social scientists, some of whom had previously drawn attention to the 'problem' of differential fertility among social groups, discovered 'the population explosion' in the Third World and argued that economic development compatible with the 'free enterprise system' might be impossible if means were not found to curb birth rates. The leader of this group was Princeton demographer Frank Notestein, who took leave from the Office of Population Research in 1959 to assume the presidency of the Population Council. This is a research organization founded by John D. Rockefeller, III, in 1952 as an outgrowth of his interest in foreign affairs, public health, and the spectre raised by Notestein and others of widespread social instability and economic failure bred by 'the population explosion' ([45], pp. 281–288).

While Population Council-sponsored research was convincing academics and political influentials of the dangers posed by rapid population growth, Notestein had become convinced that population control programs based on conventional contraceptive technology were futile. Believing that the future of the free world might be at stake, he remembered, "I've never been in another situation in my life that made me feel so helpless" ([45], p. 305) This sense of urgency led to reevaluation of a contraceptive that had been in disrepute since the nineteenth century: the intrauterine device (IUD).

In the mid-nineteenth century, when physicians first began to venture into the vagina as a matter of routine, an amazing variety of pessaries were developed for manipulation of the uterus. Among these were 'stem pessaries' that consisted of a tube fitted through the cervical canal into the uterus, with a round plate or button remaining outside the uterus against the cervix. Some physicians began touting these devices as contraceptives, but their use led to many serious infections, and they became associated with quackery. In 1930 a German gynecologist, Ernst Gräfenberg, reported on his experiments with a true intra-uterine contraceptive device, a ring of silk gut and silver wire that was placed entirely inside the uterus, and claimed remarkable success in a series of 1,000 patients. Painful dilation of the cervix was required to insert Grafenberg's ring, however, and the vast majority of physicians remained hostile toward this kind of experimentation because of justified fear of pelvic inflamatory disease and because contraception was a practice that lacked the social justification needed to warrant such risk. Nevertheless, a small number of gynecologists in the United States, some of whom were German emigrés, continued to experiment with versions of this device ([45], pp. 274–276, 305–307).

Alan F. Guttmacher, chief of obstetrics at New York's Mount Sinai Hospital, was a long-time advocate of population control and a member of the medical advisory committee of the Population Council. When a Berlin-trained colleague approached him in 1958 with the suggestion that a better IUD was possible, Guttmacher listened. Plastic made it possible to avoid dilation of the cervix by stretching a moulded coil onto a thin linear inserter; antibiotics had eased the pervasive medical anxiety over inducing pelvic inflamatory disease; the Population Council was winning an ever larger audience for the idea that a demographic emergency existed in the Third World. Under the leadership of Guttmacher and Notestein, the Population Council invested more than $2.5 million in the clinical testing, improvement and statistical evaluation of the IUD in the early 1960s. By 1967 Council members were confident that it was possible to curb birth rates in such places as South Korea, Taiwan, and Pakistan through family planning programs in which the IUD was the principal contraceptive means.

The second major advance in contraceptive technology of the 1960's was the 'anovulant' pill based on synthetic analogues of the steroid hormones progesterone and estrogen. When Gregory Pincus, the biologist who is generally credited as 'the father of the Pill,' reviewed the factors that drew him into the search for a better contraceptive, he cited "(a) a visit from Mrs. Margaret Sanger in 1951 and (b) the emergence of the appreciation of the importance of the 'population explosion'"([43], pp. 5–6). Frank Notestein and Alan Guttmacher began with a social concern and sought a solution through technological innovation that had previously seemed unnecessary, if not unethical. In the same way, Pincus began his search for a new contraceptive, in part because feminists urged him to do so and promised to pay him well for his efforts, and in part because population control was becoming a legitimate, and even glamorous, field of research. The realization of Sanger's dream of a female-controlled method that would be completely divorced from coitus could only be achieved when her feminist motives were bolstered by new economic and political sanctions for birth control ([45], pp. 376–399, 334–345).

Pincus was a scientific entrepreneur par excellence ([45], pp. 346–366). Carl Djerassi and his team of chemists at Syntex provided Pincus with the key drug he needed when they synthesized the first orally active progestin from relatively inexpensive vegetable sources in 1951 ([13], pp. 245–248). The rationale for Djerassi's new molecule was cancer therapy, however, and there was no guarantee that this wonder drug would be translated into a marketable contraceptive. Pincus had to overcome much resistance and skepticism on his way to winning acceptance for oral contraception. He had to win over critics within J. D.

Searle and Company, his commercial sponsor, who argued that one could never justify interfering with basic reproductive mechanisms simply for the sake of easier contraception. Pincus had to enlist clinicians and their patients to test powerful drugs that had many side effects, and finally to overcome resistance in the Food and Drug Administration (FDA) to licensing the massive dosing of healthy women with synthetic hormones. He was able to do these things because of major changes in attitudes toward sexuality and population growth. It is possible that oral contraceptives never would have gotten onto the market if the FDA had not approved them in 1960, because of the Thalidomide scandal and other events which soon changed the regulatory atmosphere in the FDA and made the public anxious about the drug's side effects [37].

The claim is often made that the new and 'scientific' pill and IUD had a 'revolutionary' impact on sexual behavior and values, but these innovations should be understood as responses to a changing cultural environment rather than as major causes of change. Americans were successful contraceptors before 1960. After 1960 doctors in birth control clinics often encountered 'hurting diaphragm syndrome' among women who believed their well-being required a pill, but their parents had controlled their fertility with condoms, diaphragms, and douches. Ironically, the 'use effectiveness' of the pill has not been higher among many groups than that of conventional methods ([45], pp. 365–366, 375–376). The motivation of the contraceptor remained the key factor in the effectiveness of even a magic bullet.

SUMMARY

The history of contraceptive practices in the United States is a small part of a larger story that begins with the rise of the companionate family based on romantic love and continues today with the emergence of 'the universal marketplace' in which the working mother is normative, and ever more human needs are satisfied through market transactions. The most important changes in the history of contraceptive practices did not involve scientific discoveries or technological innovations but shifts in social values and expectations. Before the 1960s, Margaret Sanger and a few feminist allies were almost alone in their liberal belief that reproductive decisions should be left to individual women, and in Sanger's case we should not forget her glib acceptance of eugenic sterilization in the 1920s. In her efforts to promote contraceptive practice, Sanger had little choice in fellow-traveling with such eugenicists as Clarence Gamble and with the architects of 'the feminine mystique' of suburban housewifery because few took her feminist ideology seriously.

The emergence of the working mother as an essential producer in liberal capitalist society, and the redefinition of the 'population problem' set the stage for the rapid changes in the law and federal policy during the 1960s that marked the official recognition of birth control as an essential and constructive social practice. Sober academic demographers were appalled when popularizers translated their warnings about the possible consequences of rapid population growth in the Third World into Jeremiads about 'ecocatastrophe'. A new conservation movement provided a focus for a broad range of discontent in affluent Cold War America with its continuing inequities and contradictions [18]. Among the most remarkable results of the new 'ecology consciousness' were bumper stickers declaring "The Population Bomb is Everybody's Baby" and "Zero Population Growth Now".

In 1984 it was still not clear whether the ideal of individual reproductive autonomy could survive another redefinition of the population problem or whether American society could afford or was willing to let individuals manage their fertility for themselves. Despite competing demands from those who favored and those who feared population growth, however, the increasing acceptance of the idea that individuals had the right to manage their fertility according to personal interests and desires marked a dramatic change in social values. A private vice had become a public right.

Rutgers University
New Brunswick, New Jersey

BIBLIOGRAPHY

1. Barker-Benfield, G. J.: 1976, *The Horrors of the Half-Known Life: Male Attitudes Toward Women and Sexuality in Nineteenth-Century America*, Harper & Row, New York, N.Y.
2. Beebe, G.: 1942, *Contraception and Fertility in the Southern Appalachians*, Williams & Wilkins, Baltimore, Md.
3. Biller, P.: 1982, 'Birth Control in the West in the Thirteenth and Early Fourteenth Centuries', *Past and Present* **94**, 3–26.

4. Braverman, H.: 1974, *Labor and Monopoly Capitalism: The Degradation of Work in the Twentieth Century*, Monthly Review Press, New York, N.Y.
5. Bullough, V.: 1981, 'A Brief Note on Rubber Technology and Contraception: The Diaphragm and the Condom', *Technology and Culture* **22**, 104–111.
6. Cirillo, V.: 1970, 'Edward Foote's *Medical Common Sense*: An Early American Comment on Birth Control', *Journal of the History of Medicine* **25**, 341–345.
7. Cirillo, V.: 1973, 'Edward Bliss Foote: Pioneer American Advocate of Birth Control', *Bulletin of the History of Medicine* **47**, 471–479.
8. *Commonweal*, September 12, 1958, 583.
9. Connelly, M.: 1980, *The Response to Prostitution in the Progressive Era*, University of North Carolina Press, Chapel Hill, N.C.
10. Corner, G.: 1964, 'The Early History of the Oestrogenic Hormones', *Journal of Endocrinology* **31**, i–xii.
11. Degler, C.: 1980, *At Odds: Women and the Family in America from the Revolution to the Present*, Oxford University Press, New York, N.Y.
12. Dickinson, R. and Bryant, L.: 1931, *Control of Conception*, Williams & Wilkins, Baltimore, Md.
13. Djerassi, C.: 1979, *The Politics of Contraception*, Norton, New York, N.Y.
14. Editorial Staff of the Alkaloida Clinic: 1902, *Sexual Hygiene*, The Clinic Publishing Company, Chicago, Ill.
15. Filene, P.: 1976, *Him-Her Self: Sex Roles in Modern America*, New American Library, New York, N.Y.
16. Fishbein, M.: 1925, *Medical Follies*, Boni & Liveright, New York, N.Y.
17. Fisher, E.: 1979, *Woman's Creation: Sexual Evolution and the Shaping of Society*, Anchor Press/Doubleday, New York, N.Y.
18. Fleming, D.: 1972, 'Roots of the New Conservation Movement', *Perspectives in American History* **6**, 7–91.
19. Foote, E. B.: 1864, *Medical Common Sense*, The Author, New York, N.Y.
20. Ford, C.: 1945, *A Comparative Study of Human Reproduction*, Yale University Publications in Anthropology, 32, New Haven, Conn.
21. Freedman, R. et al.: 1959, *Family Planning, Sterility, and Population Growth*, McGraw-Hill, New York, N.Y.
22. Gebhard, P. H. *et al.*: 1958, *Pregnancy, Birth and Abortion*, Harper & Row, New York, N.Y.
23. Gordon, L.: 1976, *Woman's Body, Woman's Right: A Social History of Birth Control in America*, Grossman, New York, N.Y.
24. Hale, N.: 1971, *Freud and the American: The Beginnings of Psychoanalysis in the United States, 1876–1917*, Oxford University Press, New York, N.Y.
25. Hoffer, P. C. and Hull, N. E.: 1981, *Murdering Mothers: Infanticide in England and New England, 1558–1803*, New York University Press, New York, N.Y.
26. Hawthorn, G.: 1970, *The Sociology of Fertility*, London, U.K.
27. Himes, N.: 1936, *Medical History of Contraception*, Williams & Wilkins, Baltimore, Md.
28. Hunt, D.: 1970, *Parents and Children in History: The Psychology of Family Life in Early Modern France*, Basic Books, Inc., New York, N.Y.
29. Kellum, B.: 1974, 'Infanticide in England in the Later Middle Ages', *History of Childhood Quarterly* **1**, 367–388.

30. Kett, J.: 1977, *Rites of Passage: Adolescence in America*, Basic Books, Inc., New York, N.Y.
31. Kinsey, A. *et al.*: 1953, *Sexual Behavior in the Human Female*, W. B. Saunders, Philadelphia, Pa.
32. Kiser, C.: 1962, 'The Indianapolis Study of Social and Psychological Factors Affecting Fertility', in C. Kiser (ed.), *Research in Family Planning*, Princeton University press, Princeton, N.J.
33. Kopp, M.: 1933, *Birth Control in Practice*, McBride, New York, N.Y.
34. Langer, W.: 1974, 'Infanticide: A Historical Survey', *History of Childhood Quarterly* **1**, 353–366.
35. Littlewood, T.: 1977, *The Politics of Population Control*, University of Notre Dame Press, Notre Dame, Ind.
36. McCarthy, M.: 1954, *The Group*, Harcourt Brace Jovanovich, Inc., New York, N.Y.
37. McFadyen, R.: 1976, 'Thalidomide in America: A Brush with Tragedy', *Clio Medica* **11**, 79–93.
38. McLaren, A.: 1978, *Birth Control in Nineteenth-Century England*, Holmes & Meier, New York, N.Y.
39. Meeker, E.: 1972, 'The Improving Health of the United States: 1850–1915', *Explorations in Economic History* **9**, 353–373.
40. Mohr, J.: 1978, *Abortion in America: The Origins and Evolution of National Policy*, Oxford University Press, New York, N.Y.
41. Noonan, J.: 1965, *Contraception: A History of Its Treatment by the Catholic Theologians and Canonists*, Harvard University Press, Cambridge, Mass.
42. Patten, S.: 1968, *The New Basis of Civilization*, D. Fox (ed.), Harvard University Press, Cambridge, Mass.
43. Pincus, G.: 1965, *The Control of Fertility*, Academic Press Inc., New York, N.Y.
44. Piotrow, P.: 1973, *World Population Crisis: The United States Response*, Praeger, New York, N.Y.
45. Reed, J.: 1978, *From Private Vice to Public Virtue: The Birth Control Movement and American Society Since 1830*, Basic Books, Inc., New York, N.Y.
46. Reed, J.: 1979, 'Doctors, Birth Control, and Social Values: 1830–1970', in M. Vogel and C. Rosenberg (eds.), *The Therapeutic Revolution: Essays in the Social History of American Medicine*, University of Pennsylvania Press, Philadelphia, Pa.
47. Reiss, I.: 1960, *Premarital Sexual Standards in America*, Free Press, Glencoe, Ill.
48. Ryan, M.: 1975, *Womanhood in America: From Colonial Times to the Present*, Franklin Watts, New York, N.Y.
49. Shorter, E.: 1982, *A History of Women's Bodies*, Basic Books, Inc., New York, N.Y.
50. Stone, H.: 1928, 'Therapeutic Contraception', *Medical Journal and Record* **cxxvii**, 21 March 1928, 7–17.
51. Stone, L.: 1977, *The Family, Sex and Marriage in England*, 1500–1800, Harper & Row, New York, N.Y.
52. Susman, W.: 1979, ''Personality' and the Making of Twentieth Century Culture', in P. Conkin (ed.), *New Directions in American Intellectual History*, Johns Hopkins University Press, Baltimore, Md.
53. Wells, R.: 1975, 'Family History and Demographic Transition', *Journal of Social History* **9**, 1–19.

H. TRISTRAM ENGELHARDT, JR.

PERSONS, SEX, AND CONTRACEPTIVES

The history of contraception reveals a number of shifts in our appreciation of ourselves as persons. By 'appreciations of ourselves' I mean to
indicate general ways in which we understand ourselves, which general
perspectives depend on major metaphysical and moral premises concerning the human condition. Some refer to these major constellations
of metaphysical, social, and scientific assumptions as paradigms, loosely
following Thomas Kuhn [9]. One could perhaps better employ the term
used by Ludwik Fleck, thought-style or Denkstil, to identify a cluster of
directing metaphysical, evaluational, and scientific commitments, as
well as social structures, along with models as exemplars through which
a taken-for-granted structure of meaning is experienced by individuals
[3]. Here the work of phenomenologists such as Alfred Schutz can also
aid us in understanding how elements of the life world, such as views
regarding sexuality and reproduction, become constituted for us and
change, as metaphysical assumptions change [13]. We understand the
moral probity of contraception through a prism of ideas and values.

   To begin with, one must note that the moral problematic of contraception itself depends on special metaphysical, moral, and/or religious assumptions. The very notion that special moral difficulties attend
prudent rational attempts to control reproduction itself requires a
constellation of assumptions. As John Noonan has shown [10], the
Christian West was the inheritor of a number of views about the nature
and significance of human biology. These views interplayed in ways that
created what was for over a millennium the received Western understanding of sexuality and of the authority to control sexuality. First
among these was a view indebted to Greek sources, including the
writings of Aristotle, which portrayed the human mind as able to know
essences in a fashion that our 20th century lights of reason do not
presume. As Marjorie Grene once argued on a similar point [5], there is
no *nous*, there is no faculty of the human mind capable of disclosing a
strictly delimited genus from which one can derive necessary, universal
first principles of intelligibility including an essential appreciation of the
significance of sexuality for a particular species – in this case humans.

39

Stuart F. Spicker, William B. Bondeson, and H. Tristram Engelhardt, Jr.
The Contraceptive Ethos, 39–45.

We inherited as well from the Stoics a view that one could intellectually discern the laws of nature to which prudent men and women ought to submit in order best to advantage their fortunes. These natural laws were held to include a *jus gentium* [a law of nations or law of the world] as being the law observed by all mankind [4]. Finally, the Christian worldview added the notion that it would be not only imprudent but offensive to the Deity to violate natural law. Thus in the words of Pius XI in his Encyclical *Casti Connubii*, "no reason, however grave, may be put forward by which anything intrinsically against nature [here, artificial birth control] may become conformable to nature and morally good" ([12], p. 92, Sec. 54). In fact, the Christian worldview that still underlies many of our suppositions not only took for granted that one could discover the natural law, including the general purposes of the human body, but that violation of that law, or subversion of those purposes, is a violation of the wishes of the Deity. In addition, the natural law was seen as providing grounds for civil authority intervening with force. Thus Pius XI also supported civil laws against adultery and birth control ([12] Sec. 73 and 124).

As James Reed indicates, our modern use of contraception presupposes that (a) there is nothing unnatural, in the sense of morally improper, in the use of contraception, and (b) civil authority does not have a moral warrant to constrain the reproductive interests and desires of individual men and women. We who live after the collapse of the Christian synthesis, and in particular after Charles Darwin, have a different understanding of the significance of the specific, peculiar characteristics of humans, including human sexuality. Natural selection has produced us as individuals adapted to environments in which we no longer live. Far from seeing the deliverances of evolution as normative, the 'natural laws of sexuality' can at best be appreciated as usually functional and benign insofar as our current environments do not dramatically diverge from those in which the patterns in question evolved, and insofar as our goals are not too distant from the 'goals' of maximizing inclusive reproductive fitness. As Donald Symon has argued, our present cluster of sexual and aggressive impulses is at best only in part congruent with our prevailing moral judgments and interests [14].

Such appreciations of human sexuality force us to recognize that we are persons judging the moral significance and usefulness of the impulses and capacities that evolution has given us. John Noonan discerns a reflection of this view, surely within constraints, in some current Roman Catholic thought. We view ourselves across a distance that looms between us as persons and the particular characteristics of our human nature, including our sexual nature. The distance between us as persons and our human nature as the deliverance of evolution invites us to restructure and manipulate that nature to meet goals chosen by us as persons. The blind, uncontrolled outcomes of reproductive acts are then morally open to manipulation through contraception and sterilization. It becomes 'natural' for us as persons to view sexuality as an opportunity alternatively for reproduction, social bonding, or recreation. In fact, it becomes quite difficult for us even to appreciate why it would be unnatural in a moral sense to use contraception to meet personal goals or to manipulate reproductive processes so as to separate the reproductive elements of sexuality from the social and recreational.

To underscore the conceptual distance between those who approve of and those who condemn contraception as unnatural, one need but read some legal codes bearing on unnatural acts. Consider the code of Virginia, which, in Section 81.2–361, included under the title 'Crimes Against Nature' carnally knowing an individual "by or with the mouth". Given the widespread peaceable indulgence in oral intercourse by males and females, married and unmarried, it is difficult for most to appreciate why such should be considered a felony.[1] The moral premises that sustained this code were similar to those that sustained much opposition to contraception. We have experienced a major abandonment of traditional metaphysical understandings and their associated moral viewpoints, which could provide generally, as *Casti Connubii* [12] and *Humanae Vitae* [11] attempted, a successful, rational argument to enforce a link between sexual love and procreation. It is no longer generally taken to be rationally demonstrable that there is a design in nature that would make acts of contraception immoral. It has become implausible that human actions should be measured against intrinsic natural laws, and more plausible that nature should be judged in terms of human goals and desires. That part of the Christian understanding of reproduction and contraception that depended not on revealed Christian scripture or tradition, but rather on philosophical-scientific argument has largely collapsed.

As Reed's article suggests, the absence of convincing natural law arguments to support civil authority controlling sexuality did not bar the entrance of the state into attempts to control reproduction. Utilitarian arguments concerning the general welfare of communities or regarding particular national policies have unfortunately been employed as an excuse for the use of state force in controlling individual sexual choices. Thus, as the view collapsed that one was constrained when engaging in sex not to thwart the reproductive consequences of sexuality in order to fulfill the requirements of the Diety, arguments were forwarded for one to reproduce in order to meet the needs of national policy, a view also seen in ancient times. What has marked the recent experience has been a recognition not only of the impossibility of establishing through general reasoning the wishes of the Diety in this matter, but the equal impossibility of establishing a moral basis for civil authority to regulate private sexual activities as well [1]. Views regarding the moral probity of contraception have become private in a way that does not discount the truth of special religious claims or the allowability of peaceably pursued political goals regarding reproduction.

The failure of arguments to establish particular sexual practices, including contraception, as unnatural in a morally normative sense, as well as the failure to secure moral authority for the state to constrain individuals to reproduce on behalf of the state, has led to a major cultural revision of the significance of sexuality. The result, however, has not been to do away with moral responsibility in reproduction. In fact, the availability of contraception has increased such responsibility. Since the production of children has a major and direct impact on others (1) through producing unconsenting third parties (children) and (2) through imposing costs on others who may need to support the third parties produced, and since such production of children can now be fairly easily avoided, the moral responsibility of those who would have children is underscored. It becomes much more difficult to establish the right to reproduce than the right to engage in peaceable, social, or recreational sex. Given the availability of effective contraception, and given the impact of reproduction on third parties, the restrictions of the People's Republic of China on individual reproductive decisions be-come more plausible. They can be understood, for example, as a form of theft from the commons, since excessive reproduction creates de-mands on commonly held goods in a way that affects the rights of other parties in those goods to which they also have a claim. Reproductive sexuality is thus freighted with responsibilities. It is easier to secure the argument that producing an extra child takes from the resources of others to which they have a claim, than it is to secure the proposition that fornication injures the rights of those not directly involved in the tryst, including the state. Other possible moral problems, even if they have not been generally translated into legal problems, have already been suggested by tort-for-wrongful-life suits in which children have sued for having been conceived or brought to term in circumstances that have led them to be born with physical, moral, or social handicaps [7].

In summary, children as a result are no longer simply seen as gifts of God. They have become the products of human choice for which reproducing individuals are responsible for their number, kind, and quality. Because of the availability not only of contraception and sterilization, but also of genetic counseling, prenatal diagnosis, and abortion, the sphere of human responsibility in the area of reproduction has been startlingly expanded [2].

But contraception not only expands human reproductive responsibilities. It makes possible a nuanced responsibility for fashioning the significance of social and recreational sex. This point has been suggested both by John Noonan and James Reed. Given our capacity to separate the social and recreational aspects of sexuality from the reproductive aspect of sexuality, we must now choose the significance we want from social and recreational sexuality. Contraception secures the possibility of various sexual lifestyles, including those of dedicated monogamy, while controlling the consequences to future children, career choices, or other individuals to whom one is committed. It must be underscored that contraception should not be seen in terms of sexual license but rather in terms of rational planning and the structuring of a life style built around carefully chosen goals for one's mate, one's children, and oneself. Contraception underscores the rational fashioning of sexual life styles.

Insofar as the choice of a sexual life style does not collide with the hard core of morality, as does using unconsented-to force against the innocent, it will be difficult to come to definitive, clear moral conclusions [1]. Moral goods will be at stake, not simply aesthetic goods, but there will not be definitive moral answers. Even after one has secured by some Kantian argument the proposition that one must keep promises, one needs to decide what promises one ought to make. The decisions to pursue a career and a monogamous marriage, or to be a sexually active single, are choices that now, given the availability of contraception, can be more easily pursued with the consent of all those directly involved. Individuals must now face a moral choice that is analogous to the choice of an artist. They must choose among alternative possibilities for fashioning the good life in the sense of a life filled with the richness of human possibilities. Contraception has separated the hard-core moral concerns of not injuring unconsenting others from the softer moral concerns of fashioning a particular vision of the good life and of the beautiful life.

It is tempting to reconstrue John Noonan's final remarks regarding balancing values in this light. The virtue of *sophrosyne* is unlike to give concrete guidance, though it may provide some regulative assistance reminding us of the ideal of compassing as many goods within as much unity as possible. We are left with little rational guidance for the difficult choices that endow our lives with content and meaning. Here Stanley Hauerwas's arguments concerning the role of moral stories are helpful [6]. We must choose among competing possibilities for our lives. One commits oneself to a tradition without decisive moral arguments. So, too, one commits oneself to a particular sexual lifestyle with its special virtues and shortcomings.

It is here that recent advances in contraception have had their influence. Consider the extent to which modern effective contraception allows each member of a couple to engage full time in the workplace and decide mutually when they will have their children with minimum anxiety about unplanned pregnancies and disruptions in life plan. Or, consider the lifestyle of the single, sexually active woman engaged full time in the workplace, who wishes never to have a child. Technology, spawned for various motives, allows styles of sexuality not available in its absence. Making love with cheap and highly reliable contraception is different from realizing contraception through engaging only in oral and anal intercourse, or with means of dubious efficacy. The kinds of contraceptives available currently, and our understanding of their actions and efficacies, give a sense of bodily control not available until recently. The availability of effective contraception has thus accentuated the notion of the human body as an object to be manipulated by humans for human goals. Contraception is thus to be understood within the general development of technology, and of medical technology in particular, which has made us an object for our own interventions.

The history of contraception is the history not only of technical advance and the collapse of neo-Aristotelian metaphysical and moral assumptions. It is also the history of the recognition of the special moral/aesthetic tasks of individuals to fashion meaning for their lives, and for communities with the grace of God or through the gift of history to offer the possibility of reproduction with meaning, reaching beyond the lives of individuals. Such is for persons and communities in the modern world an inescapable destiny.

Center for Ethics, Medicine, and Public Issues
Baylor College of Medicine
Houston, Texas

NOTE

[1] A number of recent surveys have shown the considerable frequency of oral intercourse. See, for example, [7].

BIBLIOGRAPHY

1. Engelhardt, H. T., Jr.: 1986, *The Foundations of Bioethics*, Oxford University Press, New York.
2. Engelhardt, H. T., Jr.: 1985, 'Current Controversies in Obstetrics', *American Journal of Obstetrics and Gynecology* **151** (February 1), 313–318.
3. Fleck, Ludwik: 1935, *Entstehung und Entwicklung einer wissenschaftlichen Tatsache*, Benno Schwabe, Basel.
4. Gaius: 1976, *The Institutes of Gaius, Part I*, Oxford, trans. F. De Zulueta, Clarendon Press, Oxford, p. 1.
5. Grene, M.: 1979, 'Comments on Pellegrino's "Anatomy of Clinical Judgment"', in H. T. Engelhardt, Jr., S. F. Spicker, and B. Towers (eds.), *Clinical Judgment: A Critical Appraisal*, D. Reidel Publ. Co., Dordrecht, Holland, pp. 195–197.
6. Hauerwas, S.: 1981, *A Community of Character*, University of Notre Dame Press, Notre Dame, Indiana.
7. Holder, A.: 1981, 'Is Existence Ever an Injury? The Wrongful Life Cases', in S. F. Spicker, J. M. Healey, and H. T. Engelhardt, Jr. (eds.), *The Law-Medicine Relation: A Philosophical Exploration*, D. Reidel Publ. Co., Dordrecht, Holland, pp. 225–239.
8. Hunt, M.: 1974, *Sexual Behavior in the 1970's*, Playboy Press, Chicago, Illinois.
9. Kuhn, T.: 1962, *The Structure of Scientific Revolutions*, University of Chicago Press, Chicago, Illinois.
10. Noonan, J. T., Jr.: 1966, *Contraception*, Belknap Press, Cambridge, Massachusetts.
11. Pope Paul VI: 1968, *Humanae Vitae*, Rome.
12. Pope Pius XI: 1930, *Casti Connubii*, Rome.
13. Schutz, A. and Luckmann T.: 1973, *The Structures of the Life-World*, trans. Richard M. Zaner and H. Tristram Engelhardt, Jr., Northwestern University Press, Evanston, Illinois.
14. Symons, D.: 1979, *The Evolution of Human Sexuality*, Oxford University Press, Oxford, United Kingdom.

SECTION II

IS THERE A FUNDAMENTAL RIGHT TO REPRODUCE OR CONTROL REPRODUCTION?

TRENDS AND TRENDINESS IN POPULATION STUDIES

Like a blob of ketchup on a party dress, hysteria has long formed a small but undeniable stain on the fabric of American life. One thinks first, perhaps, of the Salem witch trials or of the strange fruit of lynch victims hanging from poplar trees. And then one comforts himself by recalling that these events occurred long ago in more ignorant times. Surely, in our age of science, such hysteria would be impossible.

But suppose, one asks, that scientists join in the hysteria, and, like some old Massachusetts preachers and Southern sheriffs, lend it their authority? And so it was in the late 1960s and early '70s, as numerous scientists and their disciples hectored the public in the media and the classroom with overpopulation scenarios that could frighten one to celibacy, if not to sterility. Even rhetoric changed, as population 'growth' turned to 'boom' and then to 'explosion' and finally (and most sinister) to 'bomb'. The population would not be the target of a bomb; the population would, in its destructiveness, *be* a bomb. A Stanford biologist began his best selling book of that title with the announcement:

The battle to feed all humanity is over. In the 1970s the world will undergo famines – hundreds of millions of people are going to starve to death [6].

Meanwhile, another popular book concluded that India 'can't be saved' [12]. Similar statements multiplied, much as population problems were supposed to.

It is easy to trace the origins of this concern. In 1798 the dour English clergyman, Thomas Malthus, warned in his famous *Essay on Population* that population would grow exponentially, while its means of subsistence would grow only arithmetically. The average consumer's share, there-fore, would progressively shrink, as total output could not keep pace and increasing amounts had to be invested in capital items in a vain attempt to maintain the status quo. Similarly, the average worker's productivity, reflecting a progressively smaller portion of capital resour-ces, would shrink, too. Only pestilence, famine, war – or moral restraint or certain vices – could check the catastrophic surplus of people.

Oddly enough, the kind of population growth that exercised Malthus

Stuart F. Spicker, William B. Bondeson, and H. Tristram Engelhardt, Jr.
The Contraceptive Ethos, 49–57.

was a relatively recent phenomenon. Prior to about 1650, the natural increase – that is, the excess of births over deaths – had been about 0.05% per year for nearly two thousand years. From 1650 to 1950, the rate of natural increase proceeded at about 0.5%; and since 1950, this rate has more than tripled. Put differently, humanity had grown only to some 600 million by 1650, but reached one billion in 1850, two billion in 1930, three billion in 1960, four billion in 1974, and five billion in 1986. The main cause of the burgeoning natural increase has been a steady and marked decline in death rates, especially infant mortality, due to advances in nutrition, sanitation, and medicine; birth rates have generally fallen, too, but by a far smaller amount.

Today, however, population alarms are likely to strike Americans as quaint anachronisms, like the peace sign or the Cadillac tail fin. Hysteria, like most things, is prone to fashion, and after a while other causes displaced overpopulation. Moreover, it has become common knowledge that, though America's population continues to grow, its fertility rate has fallen significantly below the replacement level. Also below are Spain, Australia, New Zealand, Switzerland, France, the United Kingdom, Norway, Canada, Sweden, Japan, Belgium, Austria, Italy, Luxembourg, the Netherlands, Denmark, and the Federal Republic of Germany – virtually, the entire Western world plus its most important Asian partner. If this pattern persists, which is uncertain, in about twenty-five years the total population of these nations will begin a steep decline. As far as the West is concerned, the population bomb has proved to be a dud.[1]

Even duds, however, can have consequences, and so it may be useful to speculate on some of the more important results of the West's having learned the contraceptive lesson perhaps too well.

First, consider the consequences within Western nations. The best known is the rising mean age of the population, widely known as the 'graying of society'. Positively, this may mean a decline in certain anti-social, youth oriented behaviors (like violent crime) and a work force that is more mature, experienced, and reliable. Negatively, however, it may mean a loss in vitality and innovation – though this has certainly not been true of Japan or the FRG – and a higher proportion of unproductive persons requiring vast expenditures in the form of health care, pensions, and so forth.[2] The 2.6 million Americans age eighty-five and over are expected to reach thirteen million by 2040. Generational conflict, featuring a declining proportion of working age taxpayers pitted against a rising proportion of elderly 'tax eaters', may well break out into the open; when envy and resentment battle a sense of vulnerability and entitlement for huge chunks of the gross domestic product, civility even within families may be overwhelmed by events. An older workforce, moreover, will likely be a workforce committed to security before all else. This may reduce the risk taking that underpins much of the technical and entrepreneurial progress on which higher Western living standards have been built, as well as strengthen demands for protectionism and other costly anti-competitive policies. It may also further rigidify class systems and impede social mobility.

An almost equally well known change has been the movement of women from the home to the workforce. This movement, made possible by later marriages and fewer children and made necessary by an urge to raise family living standards in a period of flat real personal income levels, is by now a settled fact. It can only increase in the future. Positively, it may mean much greater opportunities for women and greater productivity for the society, but the impact of altered child rearing patterns may not always benefit the children, and may even represent a cutback in human capital investment.

There are also – to put it in the most polite terms – cultural implications of the decline in fertility. For if a society's fertility declines, it does not decline for all segments equally – indeed, some segments will not decline at all. In general, the segments whose fertility levels remain above average are the least well off, whether measured in terms of income, education, occupation, or ethnic status. They would include the poorer blacks and hispanics in the United States, for example, or the poorer Arabs in Israel or, for that matter, the poorer central Asians in the Soviet Union. In such a situation, the dominant culture (or portions of it) may feel its primacy threatened. For from its point of view, the problem is not that society's fertility rate is declining, but that the rates of the wrong groups are declining. What can the dominant culture do about the trend? By various bonus and other arrangements, of course, governments can seek to boost fertility rates, and there is always the old standby of exhortation to virtue. No government approaches, however, have proved particularly successful, especially among the more advantaged strata. Even East Germany, which spends fully three percent of its GDP on pro-natal policies and does not worry over much about domestic opponents, has achieved only a very modest return on its massive investment.

Another means of trying to keep the dominant group dominant is to attempt to lower fertility rates among those considered the peril. This can be accomplished either through inducement (e.g., offering bonuses for sterilization) or outright coercion. Frequently, eugenic rationales are given for such proposals, though they are far more important as justification than as motivation. A religious/cultural rationale is provided by Rabbi Meir Kahane, who, stressing the higher rate of natural increase among Arabs, contends that Arabs will eventually outnumber Jews in Israel, thereby transforming it from a Zionist state to something else. The only way to preserve its unique character and function, he asserts, is to expel the Arabs.[3]

Second, consider the consequences of low rates of natural increase in the West for the entire world. It is necessary to understand, in this regard, that the low rates in the industrialized so-called First World contrast with the moderately rising rates in the Soviet dominated Second World and the still higher rates in the lesser developed Third World. Thus, the First World's share of the earth's total population has fallen from twenty-six percent in 1950 to fifteen percent today and is forecasted to drop to a mere nine percent by 2025. Can the First World retain its premier position, politically, economically, and militarily, under such circumstances?

Of course, sheer numbers cannot be determinant. Technology, organization, and dozens of other factors, tangible and intangible, can be cumulatively decisive. Britain was very far from the largest country when the sun never set on its empire, and today the United States (and the Soviet Union) are not the most populous.

On the other hand, an aging population preoccupied with security and consumption may lose something in vitality, ingenuity, and hunger for success, and the technological and other means for overcoming its numerical disadvantage may no longer come so routinely. The First World may also, by dint of its shrinking vis-à-vis the Third World, be less able to influence events there. And while the First World's record in this regard leaves a great deal to be desired, there can be little doubt that it has been one of the chief causes of progress there: the Third World has drawn on First World political, economic, and social ideas; it has utilized First World technology in agriculture, pharmaceuticals, transportation, and much, much else; and it has employed large numbers of its people, generally at higher wages than had previously prevailed, working for First World corporations. Whether all these – and the veritable revolutions that they have wrought – can continue unabated as the earth's proportion of First World people declines may prove one of the more interesting questions with which the next century must grapple.

There is also, of course, the question as to whether population growth is the road to disaster. Malthus and his followers, old and new, believe that it is. But surely there is reason to doubt it. The world, after all, is far more populous today than ever before and also far more prosperous, even the Third World [7, 13, 10]. Increasingly, as a consequence, analysts are beginning to see population growth not as a liability, but also as an asset. For Malthus, as a pre-modern, seriously neglected humanity's capacity to adapt by accumulating knowledge and utilizing it in all kinds of productive innovations. Thus, the predicted Asian famines of the 1970s and '80s have become food surpluses, as increasing market reliance and the 'green revolution' have produced results that earlier alarmists could scarcely have imagined.

Also conflating Malthus is the concept of demographic transition. Originated by Thompson in 1929 [14] and subsequently criticized and revised by a number of demographers [4, 1], the concept holds that societies pass through a series of stages: first, the high birth rate is offset by a high death rate, so that the natural increase is very low; then, though the birth rate persists, the death rate declines slowly and then substantially, producing a high natural increase; next, the birth rate drops, approaching the death rate, eventually yielding an equilibrium; finally, the birth rate dips below the death rate, generating an absolute decline. Population growth, in sum, is not limited only by the apocalyptic forces that Malthus identified, but, in a sense may be self-limiting.

The Reagan administration, often attacked for pandering to its right wing supporters by cutting funding for world population control efforts, has allied itself with adherents to the concept of demographic transition. From their perspective, the traditional view that population control must proceed modernization and development ignores the fact that modernization and development are themselves principal causes of population control. Poor Third World peasants, that is, may desire large families for rational reasons: to help support the family, to provide security for parents in their old age, as insurance in the case of the early death of other children, and as a source of pleasure and fulfillment in a grim and tedious life. Modernization and development, however, undercut these motivations, in addition to providing readier access to contraception. Of course, the demographic transition concept is a general tendency rather than an iron law, but Reagan officials have seized on it to support their view that the Third World should emphasize modernization and development rather than population control as its top priority.

Ethical concerns over population tend to cluster about two issues: distributive justice and coercion versus freedom. Population policies centering on financial deprivations, for example, would clearly raise distributive justice concerns; the policies' impact would most heavily be felt upon those with the least money. Similarly, coercion is involved in such proposals as requiring an abortion when the mother is unwed [5], or in Sanjay Gandhi's compulsory sterilization efforts in India, or the anti-natal policies of China [11], where the alleged social necessity of reducing the fertility rate may collide with the traditional freedom to bear children [2, 8]. In such situations, one may either debate which of the competing claims weighs heavier in the balance or state that his value is so important that it obviates the requirement to weigh. This, however, hardly settles things. The problem with weighing competing claims is that there is no objective means of determining which claims are to be weighed or which is heavier; metaphorically comparing ethical abstractions with weights on a scale cannot negate the subjective, ultimately arbitrary nature of the decision. Similarly, declaring that (say) species survival absolutely bars large families or that reproductive autonomy bars any role for public policy are merely examples of assertions in search of arguments.

The effect of recent demographic developments has greatly complicated the discussion. If the alarmists had been correct and doomsday was nigh, many responses, including compulsory birth control [6], might find backers. An end as terrible as was forecast will justify a very wide range of means. Today, on the other hand, it is hard to be confident either that population will forever increases exponentially or even that sizable population growth is incompatible with rising living standards. Far reaching, coercive proposals, therefore, seem much harder to defend.

This is not to argue that the privateness of sexual relations necessarily excludes a governmental role. On the contrary, though making babies may be a private matter, the babies themselves have major and obvious public implications; as consumers and producers, they will make innumerable claims on their fellow citizens.

It is, however, to argue that the public policy toward reproduction should be justified by some compelling societal interest that cannot be served in a less intrusive fashion. This is true because the very privateness of sex invites heavily handed policy responses; subtle approaches are too easily evaded. Even persons hired as mere counselors may – perhaps with the best of intentions – act as regulators [9]. The temptation to regulate aggressively, therefore, may be ever present, and for that reason, should not be permitted easily.

Before closing, two important caveats, obvious and for that reason too often ignored, must be set down.

One caveat is that the future is uncertain. Projections are not predictions, and the past is littered with erroneous forecasts. The population bomb types in the '60s and '70s certainly misstated the problem. And, on the other side, following the low fertility years of the Depression and the Second World War, the U.S. Census Bureau utterly failed to foresee the great baby boom of the '40s, '50s, and early '60s; in fact, it saw a population peaking at about 165 million in 1990, a shortfall of some seventy-five to eighty million persons. To those experiencing them, trends always seem destined to go on forever, but it is not unknown for hindsight to disclose a pendulum swinging back in what had seemed an impossible direction.

Having said that, however, it appears unlikely that current low Western fertility rates will radically change soon. The main reason is that the rates are not perceived as forced on women, as were, say, the low rates of the '30s, when hard times and bleak prospects often made large families seem a quixotic choice. Today, early and large families are seen as costly in another sense: they deprive women of grand new opportunities, frequently economic opportunities. Nor, with more permissive mores and more effective contraception technology, does a decision against children or even marriage imply a decision against sexual activity or even cohabitation. Unless women become deliberated, unless real wages rise so quickly that second incomes become superfluous, unless puritanism recaptures popular morality, unless contraceptive technology collapses – unless these stunning developments come to pass, it is hard to see how baby boom fertility rates can return.

A second caveat is that just as fertility rates can be viewed as largely the consequences of innumerable discrete personal decisions, so, too, do policy responses to these rates represent decisions. As such, they are not only to some significant extent unpredictable; they are also subject to change, as decision makers change or change their minds. It is difficult to be certain what will be tried, what discarded, what altered, what retained; it is difficult to be certain what perceptions of reality, forecasts about the future, social and economic values, and political pressures will help to guide the process. But if prophecy is treacherous, it is some consolation to observe that this is in part due to humanity's dynamic role in shaping its own destiny.

Baruch College, (CUNY)
New York

NOTES

[1] Ironically, the decline in fertility was well underway even as the concern about over-population was peaking (see, e.g., [3] [14]).
[2] Of course, an aging society means that as expenditures on the elderly grow, those on the young shrink. Even if the two sets of expenditures were offsetting at a given point in time, however, their long term significance is very different: most of the expenditure on children (i.e., education, child care with mother or others) constitutes investment in human capital, which will be repaid many times over, while most of the expenditure on the aged is simply for present consumption.
[3] Calls for the expulsion of immigrants have, of course, been commonplace for years in Britain, France, the FRG, and elsewhere, though the reasons given ordinarily have been economic rather than political.

BIBLIOGRAPHY

1. Beaver, S. E.: 1975, *Demographic Transition Theory Reinterpreted*, Lexington Books, Lexington, Massachusetts.
2. Blake, J.: 1969, 'Population Policies for Americans: Is the Government Being Mis-led?', *Science* **164**, 522–29.
3. Bogue, D. J.: 1967, 'The End of the Population Explosion', *Public Interest*, (7) 11–20.
4. Cowgill, D. O.: 1963, 'Transition Theory as General Population Theory', *Social Forces* **41**, 270–74.
5. Davis, K.: 1967, 'Population Policy: Will Current Programs Succeed?', *Science* **158**, 730–39.
6. Ehrlich, P. R.: 1968, *The Population Bomb*, Ballentine, New York.
7. Hagen, E. E.: 1975, *The Economics of Development*, Irwin, Homewood, Illinois.
8. Hardin, G.: 1969, 'The Tragedy of the Commons', *Science* **162**, 1243–48.
9. Joffe, C.: 1987, *The Regulation of Sexuality*, Temple University Press, Philadelphia, Pennsylvania.
10. Morawetz, D.: 1978, *Twenty-Five Years of Economic Development*, Johns Hopkins Press, Baltimore, Maryland.

11. Mosher, S.: 1983, *Broken Earth*, Free Press, New York.
12. Paddock, W. and Paddock, P.: 1967, *Famine-1975!* Little, Brown & Co., Boston.
13. Simon, J. L. and Gobin, R.: 1979, 'The Relationship Between Population and Growth in LDC's', in J. L. Simon and J. de Vanzo (eds.), *Research in Population Economics*, JAI Press, Greenwich, Connecticut.
14. Thompson, W. S.: 1929, 'Population', *American Journal of Sociology* **34**, 959–975.
15. Wattenberg, B.: 1970: 'The Nonsense Explosion', *New Republic* (April 4 and 11), **162**, 18–23.

JONATHAN LIEBERSON

THE POPULATION EXPLOSION AND THE
CONTRACEPTIVE ETHOS

In the past quarter-century, population size, distribution and growth have become matters not only of dispassionate scientific analysis but also of concern to policy makers. In order to provide guidelines to population policy a good deal of effort has been expended: the United Nations has held meetings – such as the World Population Conferences in 1974 and 1984; the United Nations Fund for Population Activities has been created; national governments have set up commissions; and, finally, private foundations, universities and other institutions have devoted resources to research, training, technical assistance and the distribution of information. Most of this work has tried to define or assign the permissible limits of government intervention in population developments; much of it has been concerned with legal questions and human rights; and only a few philosophers have discussed the underlying ethical issues. It is one of the major ethical questions concerning population policy that is the assigned topic of this paper, namely whether there is a right to control reproduction in the light of population developments, and whether we have a moral responsibility to control reproduction in this context. While I am neither a demographer nor a professional ethicist, I venture to say that I do not find this question clear as it stands; however once its ambiguities and unclarities are exposed, other questions of interest may be substituted for it and discussed with profit.

There seem to be two rather large difficulties with the customary way of phrasing the ethical question of governmental intervention in population matters in order to pursue moral ends. The first concerns the interpretation of data concerning population variables like fertility and mortality, and the second has to do with the notion of 'our responsibility' to do this or that in light of these phenomena.

First, it is often assumed or suggested that population 'problems' arise and that upon reflection on these problems we bring in mortality *ab extra* in order to 'appraise' them. Is this true? I do not believe so.

Can one determine, in a value-free way, that there is a 'problem' based on the facts of contemporary population growth? Certainly there

59

Stuart F. Spicker, William B. Bondeson, and H. Tristram Engelhardt, Jr.
The Contraceptive Ethos, 59–87.
© *1987 by D. Reidel Publishing Company.*

has been an extraordinary increase in the world's population: in 1981 it was a total of four and a half billion, and recent United Nations sources claim that the world's population will reach over six billion by 2000, and perhaps nine billion by 2050; the growth rate of the world population appears to have peaked around two percent per year in the 1980's, but the yearly absolute increase in numbers continues to rise – three years ago, for example, some 75 million were added – so that the addition to the world's population between the years of 1980 and 1982 was greater than the present-day population of North American, Europe, the USSR, Japan and Oceania combined [13].

In what sense can one claim that these facts constitute a problem, a 'population explosion?' The issue is important because if there is no population explosion, the question we wish to address evaporates; if there is no population explosion, there cannot be a responsibility to control it.

One way in which we might claim that problems do or do not exist in an objective fashion, would be by appealing to a general scientific theory that could deliver such a judgment in the presence of initial conditions. Such a theory would entail judgments that a problem is or is not present in a region at a time, conjoined to other statements concerning the economic and social development of the region together with an account of the population growth rate. But is such a theory available, and if so, is it the sole one that commands assent?

There are, no doubt, many theories available, but none commands the field, as is evident from a brief survey of the different views concerning the impact population growth has upon economic and social development. Some authors have claimed that population is not a problem at all, or at any rate, not the chief villain, the latter role being reserved for 'underdevelopment' and the depletion of world resources. Others have insisted that the 'population explosion' is a false issue deliberately created by dominant countries in order to keep the less developed countries in their dependent condition. Still others believe that population growth is not problematic but is desirable because it is essential to development; a large population provides consumer demand to generate desirable economies of scale in production, lower costs of production, provides a low-cost supply of labor, and so on. Some of these thinkers have claimed that underpopulation has been responsible for the underdevelopment of arable land in large tracts of

Africa and South America. Many believe that an increase in population is desirable for military strength. The most influential of recent pro-population theorists, J. L. Simon [16], claims that population growth creates solutions to our problems of food resources and energy, and reminds us that the key to economic development is not merely re-sources and capital, but human capital, knowledge, ingenuity and industriousness; to think otherwise, he adds, is to fall prey to the fabrications of the 'population establishment' responsible for twisting facts to suit a Doomsday vision of the future.

On the other side are those who claim that population growth poses a threat to world stability. The most extreme views attribute nearly all of the world's ailments to over-population: poverty, low levels of living, poor health, malnutrition, pollution, and metropolitan concentration. Years ago, the Ehrlichs announced that world food catastrophes would occur unless sharp declines in world population growth occurred; and recently the Worldwatch Institute, headed by Lester Brown, claimed that the earth's ability to support adequate food and energy resources is becoming increasingly uncertain as world population moves toward the five billion mark, and unless there are dramatic shifts in population policy, famine and severe economic hardships cannot be avoided. According to this view, nothing short of coercive force may be sufficient to execute the appropriate population policies.

The existence of these extreme views indicates that there is no consensus on the most important question at hand, viz., the relation between population and development, and indirectly the question of whether population growth rates pose a 'problem' that must be 'solved'. No one social scientific theory rules the field; yet this is not the end of the story, for a moderate position is held by many thinkers. This position claims that demographic expansion can indeed be a drag on efforts to create a modern economy; that where economic gains might, population growth absorbs them; further, that rapid population growth prevents or hinders the absorption of population into a high-produc-tivity economy. More specifically, it is argued that rapid growth con-stricts development options, imposes new organizational demands on a society, intensifies economic, social and psychological problems asso-ciated with the various conditions of 'underdevelopment', and retards prospects for a better quality of life in the present and future. In this view, only in extreme cases does population growth serve as a direct

contributor to political and economic instability or ecological disaster; it
is not the sole cause of underdevelopment, but remains an important
factor in trying to improve the quality of life.

That no general theory governing the application of the term 'is a
problem' to population phenomena is universally accepted does not
imply that none exists or is true. Nevertheless, it seems likely that no
social scientific theory of this kind will be forthcoming. Some sociol-
ogists and demographers are accustomed to saying that whether or not a
general theory is available, we can assert that demographic factors are
important in determining human welfare, or are more important than
other factors. But few ever make clear what is meant by claiming that
population is "important" in determining national economic development or security or constitutes a strain on socialization mechanisms.
They rarely provide evidence that population is a more important
determinant of phenomenon X than factor Y in a statistical or corre-
lational sense (i.e., that X occurs more often in the presence of some
determinate values of population variables than Y). Nor do they provide evidence that population processes or factors are 'important' or
'more important' than some other factors as underlying causal mechanisms (as opposed to mere surface events). They usually do no more than
to assert an *explanatory preference*: that is, they prefer to use theories of
social change or maintenance according to which demographic processes play a deeper or more fundamental explanatory role than other
factors. Thus, we are back to square one: they are simply asserting that
population affects human welfare in this or that way because their
favorite theory, as yet insufficiently tested, or untestable, says so.
Occasionally they confuse this with the quite different claim that population is important because it is the most efficiently acted upon, easiest to
affect variable through policy.

Again, it is important to note that the absence of adequate, general
social scientific theories in this area is no proof that none exist, or that
there are not 'objective' population problems: yet it is difficult to arrive
at *a justified claim* that there is. (For what would be the basis of such a
claim if we lacked objective supporting reasons?) To be sure, it is
possible to employ a *terminology* for describing the presence of a
population problem: for example, we may say that individual decisions,
when 'integrated', produce a state of affairs that is not in the 'public
interest' and not rational from the standpoint of social rationality.
Accordingly, restrictions on individual fertility decision making would

contribute towards the provision of a public good, even if each individual has a rational ground for not cooperating. But this analysis presupposes specification of everything that is at issue: the values of individuals and the public.

The search for a value-free method of defining or identifying 'population problems' is fruitless: the articulation of such problems is not a social-scientific affair which delivers the statement of a condition to which morals are then 'applied'; it is a moral affair from the outset, presupposing moral values and ideological premises which justify and explain particular evaluative judgments about population size, structure and distribution. Presumably, choice of means to 'solve' such problems is no less saturated with ethical and moral premises.

But that population problems are intrinsically value-laden does not indicate the complexity of the process whereby they are recognized or acted upon by individuals and governments. Social problems of this kind always arise within a political setting; in a sense, a 'solution' to such problems always favors some interests over others, and constitutes a contest over the control of certain desirable resources(i.e., wealth, privilege, power, etc.). It is within a context of conflict of interests and values that population problems arise and are dealt with.

So much for the technocratic interpretation of population problems which regards their detection and appraisal as a value-free manner. The issue is important because if population problems are already moral, then the question of what we should do about them is already, in some sense, constrained by moral premises or values. If a concern for human welfare is already implicated in our definition of a population problem, then to be consistent, the same value *prima facie* is involved in our dealing with the problem. If this is so, an important feature of the morality of policies designed to affect demographic processes is revealed.

What, in general, should be done about population problems? It is a difficult question to answer. I do not know how to appraise the ethical status of population policies in general, and do not find it useful to speak of a single 'responsibility' or 'duty' to control reproduction in light of current population processes.

The question can be addressed in the following way. When it is asked what responsibility we have to control reproduction in light of the population explosion, it is really not clear whose or what responsibility is spoken of. When we speak of 'our responsibilities', who does 'our' refer to? What is meant by 'responsibility' in this context? In what role or capacity are we mentioned? As individuals? As citizens of our country? As moral agents? Is our responsibility a role, function, trust, duty, or obligation? If we have a responsibility is it one we can act upon, or do other duties conflict with it or override it? Before these questions are addressed more closely, it is important to briefly review the work that has already been accomplished in the area of population ethics to clarify this issue.

The earliest writings on the 'ethics of population' dealt with a number of issues, from the morality of parent-child relations to the ethics of migration policies, but foremost of concern in these early works was the question of the ethical status of government intervention in fertility decision making. With the 'doomsday' atmosphere of the 1960's, many authors focused upon the questions associated with government efforts to control population trends in the name of the public good, and more often than not, addressed the problem in the US setting rather than the more perplexing and complex situation in which non-democratic political structures and foreign cultural assumptions were present. Thus, the *US Commission on Population Growth and the American Future*, together with many other inquiries, confined itself to the issue of what conditions were sufficient for a democratic government, based upon the consent of the people, to intervene responsibly in the 'private' decisions of parents to have children; the answer weighed the civil and moral 'rights' of parents against the 'right' of government to promote public goods and welfare, depended upon the seriousness of the problem posed by unchecked population growth, and contained a list of the various 'basic values' the democratic governments ought to promote on behalf of the members of their states.

This was the context in which most of the discussions of population ethics took place up to the middle of the last decade. With the World Population Conference of 1974 in Bucharest, however, radical changes were introduced, not only in the manner in which the ethics of population were discussed, but even in the way the problems inherent in it were defined. There was no uniform agreement on the nature of the 'population problem' that motivated the creation of ethical guidelines to discipline the design and implementation of programs intended to alter fertility and other trends; there were voices which denied the very existence of such a problem. At least three major changes in the discussion of population ethics were prominent: (1) the relevance of the setting in which population problems (and consequently ethical considerations bearing upon these problems) had been previously discussed was challenged: the 'population problems' (if any) in countries without democratic political systems (and espousing entirely different conceptions of what is and what is not 'moral and ethical' or consistent with 'human rights' in the way of government intervention in family decision making and other private decisions) were not amenable to treatment with the distinctions and methodological categories that had been used in discussing the US example, nor was much assistance provided in such discussion by listing 'basic values', when conceptions of these values differed radically from nation to nation, either among government elites or among the population at large; (2) the proposed assimilation of efforts to alter population trends to development strategy simulated the critique of the former on grounds that had been previously confined to the latter: the 'ethics of development' was transposed to consideration of population policy; (3) the importance of political forces in defining and shaping a 'population problem' in a region as well as in creating a public appreciation for it was underscored – the 'politicization' of population problems was noted.

These changes added a new dimension to population ethics; while earlier discussions in the field were confined to ethical issues arising within one state and one political system – usually a liberal democratic one – it was urgently required to address not only earlier problems, but also the ethical issues which arose within states dominated by different political systems and also *between* states with distinct political systems, ethical traditions, and moral codes. What became important was the analysis and criticism of opposing ideologies regarding population trends and tendencies, and the development of critical instruments of analysis whereby such conflicts might be resolved.

Only in recent years has a distinctive field of inquiry denominated 'population ethics' arisen. Ideological conflict, and value conflict in general, was hitherto usually treated by political scientists, who also contributed to our understanding of the political roots of government attention to population problems, political impact of population trends, and political elements in the funding of population research. At first, ethical inquiry proper into population topics was, like the *US Commission* reports, largely analysis of basic values like 'freedom' and their application to fertility decision making. But with time, highly sophisticated philosophical work was produced-perhaps stimulated by some remarks by John Rawls in his *Theory of Justice* [14] concerning population size and utilitarian theory. A volume devoted entirely to moral issues and population policy was published recently [3], and scores of articles touching upon population matters, directly or indirectly, have been produced.

Much of this work is good. But much of it has also succumbed to one of two errors of emphasis or approach. On the one hand, we have read abstract theories and juggling of moral concepts with little relevance to ongoing policy inquiries. On the other hand, those thinkers who have avoided the first approach of deductive analyses of moral concepts then rather heavy-handedly applied to population matters, jump to the other extreme and are content to list a few 'basic values', claim they must be respected, and thus say even less than the first group of thinkers. Nearly everyone could agree that certain values are 'basic' or 'ultimate'. The difficulty is that these values shift in importance from context to context, no two of which are identical; ranking of values in a context-independent fashion is of dubious value, perhaps, but so, on the other hand, is simply mentioning them. Moreover, these values are intimately interrelated in practice: promoting one may lead to diminishing the presence of others; one cannot examine policies without reference to the total picture in which the values in question are 'realized'; a rationalization for practically any policy may rattle around in the logical space which the values define.

Neither of these extreme methods of ethical analysis seems promising. Let me therefore indicate in some detail what approach I would employ. Morality is the field of inquiry which studies *choice between conflicting values* – choice that is constrained by the claims made upon us by others. In this view, moreover, morals grow out of natural conditions, the conditions whereby human beings live with one another. As human beings, we have wants and desires and we wish to fulfill these desires; with the growth of thought, we learn to discriminate among desires: we foresee, plan and develop concepts of what is good. Out of this reflection upon the good, we hit upon objects which supply genuine and enduring fulfillment, i.e., the Good. Alongside this process, however, we live with others in society, in relations of both mutual benefit and antagonism, and relations of this kind give rise to claims and expectations. Reciprocity is demanded of us; laws, duties, and rights are born – standards which constrain our activities.

These conceptions of the Good and the Right may be amplified briefly. It is notorius that human beings have desires which clash and collide with those of others. In this fact lies the problem of what is good truly and finally, and of which institutions and patterns of life might conduce to this 'real' or 'true' Good. Perhaps the greater part of the work of ethicists in the utilitarian tradition has been devoted to articulating what precisely the Good consists of. Writers in the deontological tradition, stemming largely from Kant, have stressed law, duty, and obligation. When our personal goods conflict with those of others, we are likely to judge our own satisfactions to be of superior weight. Others, however, press their own claims upon us; they make demands and accompany these with promises and threats. These demands are generalized into laws, obligations and duties; they are what is right. Standards arise within the conflicts mentioned above, standards which regulate what we praise and blame, approve of or disapprove of, and these very standards can become the focus of debates which cause reflection upon conduct itself, upon what, in general, is good or right.

This sketch of the origins of moral conceptions does not claim that any *specific* conception of the Good or Right is to be accepted; it only offers a view as to how the ideas themselves arose, and as to how the conception of 'ethics' or 'morals', as a reflective enterprise distinct from mere custom, might have come into being.

It also explains in brief how it is that particular moral theories – such as the utilitarian or deontological theories – might have arisen. Particular contexts call out particular types of response: where the Good has been identified, but chaos reigns in practice, stress is placed on the demands of control and regulation; when individuals and groups are constrained and hampered by restrictive rules and regulations, a natural impulse is to emphasize the importance of wider goods than are currently available or recognized, and to develop standards and theories which encourage a liberation of human energies towards such goods. The effect, in what is known as 'moral theory', is the proliferation of 'moral theories', or 'moral systems'. Inevitably, such theories emphasize one or another aspect of the moral situation wherein choice must be made between conflicting goods in a manner consistent with existing claims of others. For example, a theory such as that of classical or contemporary utilitarianism, for all its sophistication, fails to do justice to our conception of respect for persons, as has been frequently pointed out [14]. The contract theories stressing individual rights, on the other side, possess difficulties of another variety (e.g., the failure to justify the origin and nature of such rights). Theories which emphasize divine commands, which are held in the greater part of the world, face another variety of problem: the justification of the metaphysical basis on which they rest. The list goes on. But that all major theories or systems of ethics should give rise to perplexities should not occasion resignation or withdrawal from morals once it is understood that such theories have a particular function to play, a function that is nevertheless not always properly recognized.

What is the occasion of theory in morals? What is the function of the numerous rules and principles in moral theory? Moral theorizing is reflective. Where the lives of individuals or groups are stable and untroubled by difficulties or problems, institutions and traditions – custom – do not need revision. But once problems arise, once conditions change, what seemed to be 'natural' needs re-examination. Action must be undertaken, yet no clear principles exist for guiding it, or else some hitherto 'external' factor enters into life which needs adjustment with existing practices. Current beliefs and institutions – family, business, industry, church, state, military – need to be altered by the efforts of individuals and groups in order to adjust to novel conditions, and existing theory does not provide guidance. The rights or wrongs of divorce, or the effects of technologies delivered by science, or economic practices, are topics which, when raised to the level of reflection as problems which demand resolution, place us in the realm of moral theorizing. We are impelled to reconsider our actions and our habits, to examine their consequences and to choose this or that course of action. The role of theory is to facilitate such action.

As stated previously, such theory as is invented is bound to be one-sided insofar as it stresses issues and factors predominant in the present scene, or rudiments and survivals of previous moral conceptions, the only conceptions at present available. This is an inevitable aspect of theory. The important point to stress is that the occasion for theory is contextual; it pertains to the specific situation under scrutiny. To be sure, elements of such theories as have been invented survive their original context; they are incorporated in later theorizing. 'Rules' of moral life are handed down: we are told to tell the truth, seek the good and secure justice. Succeeding theorists employ such directives as elements in their own work. But moral life is too complex for these 'rules' to function as *rules*; they are rather principles, elements, or factors to be taken into consideration in analyzing specific situations,

situations that involve a vast number of factors beyond those envisaged by earlier theorists. We are called upon to adjust the claims of wealth, civic duty, ecclesiastical obligations, professional life and social welfare; earlier theories, systems and rules cannot be applied directly, for they arose out of simpler problems and conditions. Rather, they are instruments for understanding various factors at work in the current scene; each may have something to offer us; none are self-contained, fully formed systems to be 'applied' deductively to contemporary conditions, but instead methods of grasping and directing these conditions.

The significant point to be stressed is that morals are not a static or fixed set of principles or rules. The fact is that the processs of theorizing adumbrated above must be done again and again: new conditions upset old habits and beliefs; we try to employ the older conceptions developed in response to older problems; we fail; we must develop new tools of analysis and new principles for adjustment of competing claims. The process may be described as that which occurs whenever reflection takes the place of custom, when customary conceptions no longer suffice. Novel conceptions and theories are developed to fit new circumstances.

We have described the conditions and processes of moral thinking that can be applied to the efforts of *individuals* to adjust to new conditions and new problems. But the concept can equally be applied to groups, cultures and societies, to 'macro ethics' – the ethics pertaining to men and women in association, for groups and societies confront problems as well. This indeed may be one way of explaining the origin of 'publics' and governments. Private transactions may or may not have indirect consequences and unintended 'spillovers'. If they do, individuals in a certain region may possess a common interest in regulating such consequences; a 'public' arises, and when it is organized so as to protect and guide the common interests of those belonging to it, a government is established. As on the individual level, social decision-making requires principles to govern the choices made by government; as on the individual level, customary methods may fail. The morality of government lies in the fact that decisions made may be better or worse, better insofar as ensuring greater freedom, liberation of individual capacities, and regulation of potentially harmful consequences to the common interest. Methods of adjustment must be devised for resolving conflicts that might arise both within and between groups or publics. The manner in which conflicts are resolved is always the same: the problem under consideration is clarified; agreements are sought on

central issues or factors pertinent to the problem; on this basis, hypo-
thetical resolutions are tried out among the competing parties; equilibrium is sought with the aid of principles and theories; agreement is
found on what to do. Any phase of this process might collapse owing to
disagreements. The issue is vastly more complicated when conflicting
cultures or societies are the parties: each side believes its beliefs and
interests are rational and objective – but objectivity is not universality –
they must *justify to each other, on the basis of common agreements*, their
proposed plans of action.

So far we have offered a sketch of morals and moral theory. Our view
is a pragmatic and contextualist one, which is opposed to rigid distinctions and priorities in the realm of moral theorizing, and which argues
for a sensitivity to values inherent in problem situations. It has been
argued that this view is defective insofar as it must accept at face value
the values of those in the problem context, that it offers no method for
resolving moral disputes except an appeal to reflection, and that it seems
to derogate the importance of fundamental moral principles. But none
of these criticisms, in fact, are correct: our view does indeed appeal to
reflection, but it is precisely for this reason that the values of those
within the problem situation must be 'accepted'; it does not regard such
acceptance as eternal, however – for such values may, should the isssue
arise, become the focus of further reflection; it does not appeal to
methods of adjusting moral conflict beyond reflection simply because it
regards reflection as a name for the methods so far devised, and it
believes that should these fail, reflection may arrive at other methods;
finally, it does not disparage familiar moral principles but rather tries to
identify their worth, and concludes that their worth does not lie with
their necessary truth, validity or their service as *rules*, but in their
capacity to serve as principles – guides to moral inquiry that have been,
and still are, useful.

Thus far, the conception of morals that controls the judgments of
population policies has been described. Associated with this view of
morals is a view of government intervention. There are two central
questions concerning the ethical status of any such intervention. The
first is: What sort of governance is in question and how are decisions
affecting its citizenry reached and implemented? This is a 'procedural'
question; it concerns how government operates, whether it takes into
account the preferences of those governed, and how it reaches decisions
and puts them into effect. The second question is: Granted some

procedure of arriving at decisions is required, what sorts of considerations have entered into the decision in question? This is a 'substantive'
question; it concerns the issue of whether the decision is right, acceptable, or 'correct'. In any discussion of government policy, these two
questions figure prominently, but they are logically independent. In my
view, we should adhere to principles of autonomy and consent in
creating and implementing any population policy, and to this end
democratic methods are the sole methods available: only in a political
system in which government rests upon freely given consent of the
governed would our ethical commitments and values be realized. This
requirement is an ideal and might exclude large portions of the political
world today; nevertheless, it seems to be a valuable ideal. It requires
active participation, free discussion and consultation in public policies,
voluntary cooperation in execution of mandates reached through democratic processes, effective mechanisms which permit prompt action
through delegated authority, intelligent methods in devising these policies,
and reliance on critical inquiry in resolving conflicts and disputes.

Of course, this process is bound in practice to encounter serious
conflicts, which brings the question of government intervention into
consideration. Should persuasion and argument fail to be effective,
coercive means might be required. No condemnation of coercion *per se*
can be made unless a specification of the end or reason for invoking it is
given, and there are countless cases of justified coercion (i.e., when a
violent mob must be restrained). There is no absolute or automatic way
to resolve the question of the justification of coercion save through
continuing judgmental review and renewing consensus on a specific
problem in a specific situation, provided procedural standards of a
democratic nature are ensured. To be sure, certain values – autonomy,
freedom, justice – must be observed as far as possible; for it is the moral
role of government to promote the welfare and, more generally, the
realization of these values for its citizens. But each situation calls for its
own specific policy: the degree of acceptable intervention, determined
by the demands of the problem and by the best available knowledge of
it, is what must be ensured. A balance between the competing claims of
the liberties and autonomy of individuals and the good of society as a
whole must be achieved.

Some qualifications must be appended to this conception of the moral
role government can play. First, granting the primacy of the democratic
procedure of institutional criticism, voluntary means should be employed

whenever possible to settle disputes or resolve differences; only if that cannot be employed or is exhausted in the presence of a serious problem threatening the maintenance of a society, should nonvoluntary means be employed. The degree of coercion brought into play should be proportional to the seriousness of the problem; employing overt violence or other potentiallly injurious coercion is not to be used before noninjurious coercion has been exhausted. Clearly there are some situations in which ethics simply does not apply at all. It is all very well to argue that universal participation in a society is ideally recommended and that institutions which fail to satisfy the desires and needs of citizens be reconstructed. But this is patently impossible in cases of emergency; in such situations we cannot afford the leisure of social reconstruction; we do not require a justification for intervening, and ordinary constraints on actions must be suspended. Accordingly, only in extraordinary circumstances is severely coercive governmental intervention in the lives of its citizens acceptable on moral grounds.

A second point concerns the increasingly employed language of 'human rights'. What are 'rights' in the foregoing conception? We have already provided the answer in part, by describing how the notion or concept of right or obligation arises under natural conditions. Individuals are not isolated, fully formed or ready-made; they are individuals, indeed, because of their relations to others. These relations are of various kinds – parent-child, employer-employee, friend-friend – but most are marked by the presence of duties that arise spontaneously and naturally, so that we say, for example, that someone who becomes a parent *by that fact* assumes various responsibilities. 'Duty' expresses such responsibilities, as do 'rights'. Right, in general, expresses the common good regulating the activities of community members. Rights are demands individuals may claim of one another, and are correlative to duties on the part of those on whom the demands are made. These relations and demands called 'rights' may vary and conflict with one another.

Many of the demands that are made on us become generalized into 'rights', which are backed by laws; they are civil or political rights which, in a given social arrangement and over the course of time, have been definitely formulated and enforced (i.e., the rights found in contract law). But, to turn to the topic that our proposed research concerns, what are 'human rights?' Clearly they are not, or not yet, legal rights; rather they are moral rights of a kind not readily identifiable. With respect to a given 'human right', a number of questions may be asked:

(1) What is a 'human right?' (Is it genuinely universal? Does its applicability vary across cultural and economic circumstances?) (2) How is it justified and on what ground? (3) What is its practical content – the conditions of its exercise? (4) What is its worth? (5) How are 'human rights' to be ranked vis-a-vis other rights, including other human rights? (6) Should conflicts arise among such rights, as occurs daily in the case of civil rights, how are such conflicts to be resolved? (7) Upon what principles of balancing or priority can we rely? (8) How is a 'human right' to be enforced? (By what agencies and under what circumstances?)

'Human rights' are morally justifiable claims made on behalf of all men and women to the enjoyment and exercise of those liberties, commodities, and services which are considered, in a specific temporal and historical context, to be inherent in our conception of what human life should be like. That is, they are normative and evaluative; they are proposals which bind relevantly placed persons and institutions to specific policies. As such, they are not founded on 'human nature' or some particular set of facts about what 'human psychology' or 'human behavior' is like, but rather are justified by reflection upon what consequences will ensue if they are pursued; they are reflected upon in light of already given values, and are never valid in isolation from a consideration of the consequences of their exercise. 'Human rights' can conflict, and this means that they must be adjusted as the specific case demands. Furthermore, their importance and worth is inextricably linked to context; although such rights do not cease to exist when incompletely ensured – an ill and malnourished man living in deplorable squalor might still have the right to free speech – they gain in worth as they are realized conjointly with other rights, whether human rights or not. We cannot judge a person to be free or in possession of his 'rights' except by judging the system of rights he enjoys, and in a specific context of resources available to him. The question of which human rights are more 'basic' than other receives an analogous reply. For human rights are interrelated in complex ways: the condition for one right may also be a right, the exercise of one right may logically necessitate the possession of other rights, and so on; to say in general that one right is to be ranked above or below another, apart from the situation in which they are present, is not possible, and much time has been wasted in trying to specify such rankings (i.e., ranking civil and political human rights above or below economic and social human rights). Moreover, the much disputed question of citing necessary and sufficient conditions under which this or that right is 'completely realized' or 'implemented' needs to be answered as follows: human rights do not come equipped with labels upon them indicating where they apply (i.e., whether they are applicable in conditions of war); efforts to cite such conditions always fall short of adequately fitting the diversity of economic and social circumstances. In general, there is no uniform answer as to when exactly human rights are 'completely realized'. Finally, which rights are 'human rights' is a question which may evolve with economic and social development and social progress, as our present century has indisputably shown.

These views differ from the prevailing view in the philosophical and legal literature of today. The major volume on population ethics written in recent years, as well as a recent volume devoted to rights (which discusses in considerable detail the ethical issues of human rights in the population context), both make strong assumptions on individual rights that conflict with ours, and thus give rise to what, on our position, are artificial problems. Rights are proliferated indiscriminately on dubious justifying premises; they are treated as ready-made labels waiting to be 'applied' or 'implemented', regardless of circumstances, or 'ranked' in some universal manner. In addition, they are rarely anchored in any identifiable political universe. This is especially true of discussions of population aid construed as a component of human rights policy.

While it is morally commendable to promote human rights, the fact is that we live in a system of nation-states governed by the principle of self-determination, an order lamentably closer to that described by Hobbes than to that of Grotius, and marked by competitive struggles for power and the realization of specific, competing values. Under these circumstances, any policies designed to promote human rights are unlikely to be effective: human rights 'violations' (or the absence of their realization or 'implementation') are usually not surface phenomena but symptoms of deep-lying flaws in the political structure of a country, flaws that would require a reshaping of that structure if violations were to be stopped. More important, the US, in the current world order, must promote a multiplicity of ends; there are other values (including peace, nonproliferation of weaponry and security considerations) which foreign policy must promote. Human rights policy, if realistic, must be balanced by consideration of these other factors and thus be extremely modest.

The prevailing tendency of current literature seems to adulterate the value of the term 'right'. As in the documents that have been concerned with human rights, produced by the United Nations in the past quarter century, it has become customary to rename what is widely described as a 'human right'.

But what are the 'rights' or 'human rights' involved in fertility, mortality and morbidity, and migration? A tremendous variety and number of such rights have been mentioned, especially when policy measures allegedly threatening them have been proposed. With regard to fertility it has been asserted that limited access to contraceptive methods or abortions and legal measures designed to affect the composition of the population by influencing family formation – such as legal limits on age of marriage, incentive and disincentive programs, pro- or anti-natalist in intent – cannot be reconciled with the 'right' of all individuals and couples to freely and responsibly choose the number and spacing of their children. Respecting mortality and morbidity, it has been said that the absence of any effective policy of reducing or eliminating the wide differentials in mortality across the world, of reducing occupational hazards and exposure to risks in the work-place, of easing escalating costs of medical treatment, of reducing infectious and parasitic diseases, involuntary sterility, subfecundity, and illegal abortions, and of providing infant care, is a 'violation' of the right to an adequate standard of living, health, work, and life itself. Regarding migration, the absence of curbs on urbanization, for example, creates problems of adjustment and maintenance of social and cultural identity for migrants, serious shortages of housing, health care, and nutrition, and is allied to increases in crime, pollution, poor transportation, the erection of squatter settlements, inner-city slums lacking even basic sanitation facilities, widespread discrimination, and other woes. On the other hand, government policies – which have ranged from fiscal and administrative schemes such as preferential tax rates, housing subsidies, relocation grants, and loans, to outright coercion and forcible movement of people and their possessions – have been asserted to violate migrants' fundamental rights to freedom of movement and of residence, to adequate housing, sanitation, vocational training, access to trade union membership, protection against discrimination and arbitrary exploitation, and other goods and services. Are these assertions correct?

The philosophical methods mentioned above would proceed by consulting some allegedly 'justified' moral theory, deriving specific rights, claimed to be held by all human beings, and then judging proposed policies as to whether they respect such rights or not. Our own view is skeptical of such a procedure. As stated previously, in our view morals are not external to the conditions under which we live, but arise from these very conditions. What is and is not 'right' or 'a right' cannot be divorced from the plural factors in a given situation or context; neither can the issue be separated from the values and beliefs of those affected. This view does not rigidly deny the existence of human rights – on the contrary, it confirms their existence – nor is it equivalent to relativism. Rather, it makes a distinction between objective and universal rights: it might be perfectly obvious to men and women in the US that freedom from 'arbitrary loss of livelihood' is a basic human right; we regard the right as an objective one; but this right is neither realized in many parts of the globe, nor recognized to be a right; in some cases, it may be believed not to be a right at all. The matter is one of justifying our view *to* others. Usual formulations of rights, i.e., the celebrated principle that all couples and individuals have the basic right to decide freely and responsibly the number and spacing of their children and to have the information, education, and means to do so, and that the responsibility of couples and individuals in the exercise of this right takes into account the needs of their living and future children and their responsibilities towards the community, are easily agreed to once it is recognized that practically any attitude towards fertility control can be sanctioned by appeal to it. Once we ask, however, which rights are involved in current developments in genetic engineering, sex predetermination, methods of genetic diagnosis, euthanasia, or the desire of migrants to be rejoined with family members, the issues are no longer so clear, whether because irreconcilable, conflicting values are present, adequate tools of ethical analysis are not available, or a host of other possibilities. But it seems clear that little progress is made by 'applying' to a complex and changing set of conditions a fixed moral system that rests on immaculate philo- sophical foundations and chains of deductive reasoning from previously justified premises. What is a 'right' is not found ready-made in such systems, but is discovered by close analysis of the situation in which the conflict of value arises.

So far we have argued the following: it is radically unclear what the conceptual and empirical relations between population processes and human welfare are, so that justified claims to this or that responsibility are uncertain. Moreover, the lack of clear responsibilities in this context renders it uncertain whether we have responsibilities of a strong kind to specifically act or set measures 'in light of the population explosion.' We have also introduced a conception of morals which excludes appeal to some of the currently fashionable devices supporting (or undermining) population policies (i.e., 'human rights'). Nor is it helpful, in this connection, to speak of population policies as endeavors to prevent people from stealing from the commons through producing more children who would consume its products. We do not live in a commons; the world is not a commons except in the minds of a few ethical philosophers.

None of this implies that there are no population problems today. Nor does it imply that there are things we ought to do for countries with serious population problems, or that we should not alert, inform and persuade the leaders of these countries to act in certain ways to promote or arrest population trends in their countries. If a population problem occurs in a region, what is an ethically acceptable way of solving it?

Population growth can really only be reduced in a few ways: by permitting mortality to rise, promoting emigration or lowering fertility, and the first two are generally regarded as unacceptable. As such, the object of most population policies of an anti-natalist kind today is restricted to one of several possible classes of measures. By 'policy' I mean an explicit attempt by a government to affect the population growth rate, not merely a cultural practice. (To be sure, the cultural milieu of any community contains practices of this kind, i.e., religious proscriptions, early marriage, practices relating to the role of women, breastfeeding practices, divorce and-remarriage arrangements, marital needs to demonstrate fecundity or virility, son preference, sex roles, etc.)

A government can (1) manipulate public and private access to methods of fertility control (i.e., limit legal access to induced abortion or to contraceptives); (2) attempt to alter the perceived socio-economic determinants of fertility behavior (i.e., literacy, infant mortality, urbanization, income level, housing, and so forth); (3) make propaganda for lowering fertility (i.e., exhorting changing family norms for reasons of collective benefit); (4) institute incentives of a positive or negative kind, immediate or remote, individual or community (i.e., direct monetary stipends, child assistance subsidies, direct monetary payments for vasectomies, deferred monetary incentives such as interest-free loans for low-income couples, or, on the anti-natalist side, schemes such as those used on the India tea estate program in which joint savings accounts were set up in the name of the company and the mother, into which the company paid a certain amount per month each month the woman was not pregnant, or mixed incentives such as those used in Singapore – maternity leave for the first two children but not for the third or later child, preference in choice of primary school limited to the first three children, increased delivery charges in public hospitals for higher birth orders, increased tax relief only for the first three children, and so on; (5) exert socio-political pressure or impose direct sanctions on fertility behavior.

It is this last category that has, of course, aroused a great deal of controversy. What is possible in this category is easily imagined: curtailed rights for those with excess children; conditional social security benefits for small families; discrimination practiced in favor of small families in housing; a set, high minimum age of marriage; marketable licenses to have children; and involuntary fertility control, such as a temporary sterilizing agent in the water supply. It is difficult to know just what has been tried in this area but it is interesting to note that policies belonging to this type have indeed been tried in the world's largest developing countries, India, China and Indonesia. For example, it is well known that during the Emergency, India conducted an intensive drive, in some states, to reduce fertility; that targets were set and district commissioners required to achieve the given targets at some career jeopardy by whatever means they could find and that these means often included exercising power over permits, licenses, school entry, appointments, and employment; that in some instances physical coercion was used, at least substantial exercise of pressure to secure candidates for sterilization.

Indonesia has in recent years organized a political bureaucratic campaign to reduce population growth through pressure exerted at the village level. According to one observer in East Java,

a strong BKKBN (National Family Planning Coordinating Board) mobilized bureaucratic resources from the governor's office right down to the thousands of hamlet heads. By decree, every public servant was ordered to promote the family planning program in every way. This included the military apparatus as well as the government civilian structure. . . . Armed with the governor's order, the BKKBN exploited this network to mobilize community acceptance of birth control. Basically, the system works as follows: Each level of government follows directions handed down from the next higher level. . . . Messages are transmitted down the chain of command within a relatively short time. A high level decision to support a program like family planning thus implies automatic support from lower levels. The system clearly works on the basis of communication and loyalty. . . . In some areas, the hamlet head daily raps a signal on a hollow wooden instrument to remind village women to take their pills [9].

In China, similar measures have been adopted. Certainly planned regulation of population growth rates has been taken in China to be part of the planned development of the economy as a whole, with intensive efforts made to promote the two-child norm. John Aird recently notes the use of coercion in this respect:

a careful reading of the descriptions of family planning work given by the Chinese media leaves little doubt that the single most important factor [in reducing population growth rates] is direct administrative pressures on individual Chinese families by family planning cadres and other officials who are themselves under pressure to achieve quick results. The pressures range from strong persuasion to outright coercion.

Elsewhere he writes,

the use of persuasion is often so aggresive that it amounts to administrative harrassment. Its methods include repeated visits by the cadres to have 'heart-to-heart talks' with reluctant couples, prescribed participation in 'discussions' designed to 'educate' them about the need to control fertility, and the 'mobilization' of women to have intrauterine rings inserted, to be sterilized, or to have unauthorized pregnancies terminated. Instances of outright physical coercion are not often described explicitly in Chinese sources, but coercive practices are often referred to obliquely as relying on 'administrative orders', resorting to 'commandism', pursuing 'indigenous policies', 'overdoing things', and so on.

Aird mentions a campaign conducted against those who illegally remove IUDs for a fee and hints that these devices are often inserted against the wishes of the women. In certain provinces of China, he continues, levies are imposed on family income for unauthorized children, with the punishment sometimes falling on the child. Reports of forced abortions and infanticide have also been made [1].

What can be said about the ethical assessment of policies such as these and more generally about policies designed to reduce fertility? In our view, the ethical acceptability of specific population policies must be ascertained by the methods of agreement outlined earlier: there is, say, a population problem perceived in a region; a problem of this kind would only arise if values were placed on the causes and consequences of population variables; these values conflict with others (i.e., it is realized that, if our knowledge base is accurate, population growth would lead to consequences that would impair the realization of other values equally cherished). Policy makers must decide upon a course of action, a policy, which respects the claims made upon government by the individuals who form the communities to be affected by these policies. To decide upon such an issue is a moral issue through and through; it may indeed be helped by taking into account the factors stressed by classical ethical theories, but taken by themselves these theories – utilitarian, contractarian and so forth – generate perplexities, so that the choice of policy is never a matter of calculation and the theories are never substitutes for sensitivity to the conflicting claims at hand. Choice of policy – that is, the moral aspects of such choice, and not the mustering of the political force necessary to put the policy into law – must proceed by discovering the basic agreements on values shared by members of the community in question; equilibrium must be created between these values and those whose realization or promotion is desirable if the policy is to be morally legitimate.

This view might be open to several misinterpretations. First, it speaks only of a method of resolving conflicts; it does not deny the possibility of enduring conflicts. Indeed, it does not deny what is evidently an important possibility, that discussion might break down and no resolution occur at all. If we assume, as we must, that other cultures and other peoples go through a process of reflection on values similar to ours, then we must acknowledge the possibility that a reflective equilibrium between our values and theirs is not possible. Secondly, it might seem that all we are arguing is a prudential point, that it is best in designing and implementing population policies to take into consideration the values of those affected by them. We hold this as a moral consideration as well.

What would be our general appraisal of the types of policies that have been mentioned? First, we should require that unless a catastrophe is present, all such policies should be based on the free consent of those affected. If this is satisfied, a broad range of interventions is ethically acceptable. (Indeed, consider the measures that are, or have been, implemented on this basis: legal requirements of monogamy, legal establishment of age at marriage, establishment of health status of partners in marriage; requirements with regard to health practices such as vaccination; limits on international emigration and immigration, and so forth.) Under ordinary circumstances, we should regard limitation of access to methods of birth control as impermissible because it impinges on the autonomy of the individual. Incentive programs pose complex difficulties. In general, positive incentives are acceptable since they increase effective liberty, provided that the individual is not deceived in taking it up, and the system of incentives itself is not discriminatory in intent. As one writer admirably put the matter:

attempting to influence a person's decision by providing an incentive to choose one alternative rather than another does not limit a person's liberty to decide, or at least does not do so in a way which per se is morally objectionable. Instead, it increases a person's liberty or freedom to choose a certain alternative by eliminating or compensating for a feature which might restrain him from choosing it. . . . Moral objections arise when incentives are offered to encourage a person to neglect or violate his duties or obligations, for example, bribes to a commissioner to rezone property. The use of coercion to discourage a person from choosing an alternative, however, does limit his liberty to decide and is per se morally objectionable [2], p. 41f.

The possible effect on innocent third parties should also be mentioned: since negative incentives penalize those who engage in fertility behavior beyond a specified limit, the possibility of disadvantages unfairly thrust upon innocents is particularly acute. The potential disadvantages fall into two groups: first, the effects of entry into a society implementing disincentives – socio-economic status, diminished housing, schooling, and general welfare affected adversely; second, psychological or internal effects in the form of intra-family reactions to innocents on the ground that they cost the family something, subsequent regret, unfair preferment, and other attitudes causing low self-esteem. Such effects may not be large in realistic disincentive programs, but they exist nevertheless and should be safeguarded against. There are clear cases (i.e., if the Nth + 1 child is deprived of public education) that must be corrected, but the multiple ramifications of the problem of innocents are so subtle and difficult to place under standardized control that they constitute a *prima facie* reason in favor of employing positive incentives in preference to disincentives. In short, the innocent party is unduly harmed by the working out of policy – and the Singapore experience has shown that that is achievable in design and in practice.

In short, positive incentives are usually permissible – provided that other means of resolving a population problem are not sufficiently effective in their absence and that those who are affected by the incentives understand and possess sufficient knowledge of the consequences of accepting them. The potentially discriminatory effects of such a program should be reduced as far as possible through adapting and readapting the design of the program to varying situations.

Finally, there is the problem, essentially administrative but evidently ethical in implication, that incentive programs lend themselves to corruption and abuse. That is possible, of course, but we must distinguish between a policy and its application. The latter may be disastrous, a gross abuse of human rights, without in the least impugning the policy itself. It is obvious that incentive programs may be abused or corrupted (as reportedly in India), but so can any policy involving monetary transfers, indeed any policy at all. But not all policies are inevitably abused to the point of ethical inadmissibility. Instead, they are usually supplemented by qualifying conditions as to the circumstances of their application, and such abuse, far from being part of the policy itself, is not even inevitable, given decent administration. Similarly, the incentive can be misused through deceit: some people accept incentives who do not intend to or cannot have children anyway. In such cases, however, the ethical onus falls on the dissemblers, not those who offer. As for politically organized peer pressure, a mixed picture emerges of the ethical acceptability of such programs. Politically organized peer pressure seems to us permissible only under certain conditions, as enumerated below.

A few preliminary points must be made. First, it is not precisely clear how to delimit such efforts from milder policies: government information, guidance, and education shade off, sometimes imperceptibly, into 'soft' then 'hard' persuasion, and that into peer pressure, either because larger and larger groups in the society accept the views being disseminated or earlier 'failures' lead governments toward stronger and stronger measures. Ordinarily, as recent discussions in our own country indicate with regard to cigarette smoking, safety belts or pollution, we do not raise special objections when government takes the role of informant, educator, or regulator – but where does that allowance end? Is it possible to set limits on this role so that government may engage in information-giving but not in generating peer pressure that is 'politically organized?' There is a difficulty at the outset in discriminating the effects of government involvement in public concerns.

Another point that is pertinent here concerns culture. We are all born into a culture that approves or condemns certain behavior. As we have noted, cultural practices are not 'policies', but are often the residue or deposit of deliberate actions undertaken by prior dominant powers. We have already noted that it is difficult to precisely pick out the effects of government involvement in public concerns, nor do we deny government a moral role. So, if we are to be consistent, we must note that much that passes for 'culturally determined' beliefs and attitudes is politically determined. Consider attitudes towards nuptiality, mortality, and other vital areas of life: many of them are the effects of prior government enactments that have crystalized cultural practices into law, that in turn reinforce or solidify the practice itself.

In order to clarify these complex issues, let us confine ourselves to a program of politically organized peer pressure deliberately designed to promote demographic goals, whether pro- or anti-natalist, whether going against the grain of cultural practices or not. The issue is to provide ethical appraisal of such a program whether or not it is appealing to the cultural heritage, is likely to be effective, and makes use of existing practices. Is there any general judgment that can be made or laid down for such an appraisal? I think not, but do suggest that there are at least three conditions that ought to be satisfied before any such program is put into effect.

The first is that owing to the real moral risks that attend the use of any such program, it ought not to be considered before every reasonable effort has been made to exhaust the possibilities of using 'softer' measures, such as purely voluntary supply programs, positive incentives, and negative incentives harmless to innocents. The reason for this is to maximally reduce the possibilities of harmful effects and to invoke policies with potentially harmful effects only if the problem under consideration is both of sufficient gravity and sufficient recalcitrance. In each such case, I would require both that softer measures be tried out or contemplated before resorting to measures that are more ethically risky, and that an official determination of serious consequences from fertility trends without further intervention be made and balanced against the consequences of using 'harsher' measures. The justification of this 'step ladder' approach will become clearer, although it seems intuitively secure on its face.

The second condition is also a matter of procedure. I would require that members of the community to be affected should be involved, whether directly or through their representatives, in an open and fair discussion as to whether to institute the program in the first place. Of course there are snags here: the form, duration, consequences, etc. of such programs are often a matter for expert judgment. But the fundamental point I wish to make is that affected citizens should, at the very least, be able to 'talk back', to be heard up the line, regarding such issues as quotas, means, time, urgency, degree, etc. – and especially in non-open societies. (The extent to which such a requirement, vague as it may be, is satisfied in China or Indonesia today, or in India during the Emergency, is a question for empirical determination. The difficulties of making such a determination are great: whether the requirement is satisfied, varies greatly in both space and time, with local circumstances and personalities, and collecting data on the matter involves finding not only responsible and accurate informants but also careful interpretation of the data received, which frequently involves conceptual issues involving local expectations, definitions, tolerances and traditions.)

The third condition follows upon the second. Not only should community members be reasonably involved in the formulation of this policy, but they should also be reasonably and adequately protected from subsequent individual dissent. Although of the greatest importance, this requirement is difficult. Furthermore, it seems to us that the most effective means of protecting this value is through consulting community members in each case in order to ascertain the most appropriate method of protection. In Indonesia, for example, colored pins on a public bulletin board do not seem excessively harmful, but marching dissidents up and down the village street in humiliation for nonconformance, does; the villagers themselves may very well see the matter differently. (This whole issue raises the profound question of 'whose ethics' are to be observed).

Given the official nature of such political organization of peer pressure, particularly in nondemocratic or non-open societies, there is obviously considerable room for abuse of this policy. This is all the more reason to insist on these conditions as safeguards. With them, however, the practice can be seen as an attempt, under difficult circumstances, to move societies ahead, guided by major reliance upon the development of community consensus – on fertility in this case – as on agriculture, schools, roads or water supply in other cases. If it can be done with due ethical regard for the community's members – in both the policy's origination and outcome – it seems ethically admissible. These three conditions do not eliminate the possibility of deleterious effects stemming from the use of such peer pressure to reduce fertility; hence, I again stress that such programs ought not be employed unless an extraordinarily serious problem is present and schemes should be devised that carry the least possible moral risk with them.

So much for the ethical appraisal of the policies mentioned above. I have no illusion that it clarifies to any considerable extent the complex ethical issues involved in population policies; I have tried only to provide an overview of the potential issues.

Even so, the most pressing issues have hardly been touched. As said earlier, it is unclear to what extent we have anything like a generic 'responsibility' in light of the 'population explosion' to take this or that action. Moreover, contrary to a celebrated remark of Robert McNamara's, I do not believe that population processes today pose a threat equal to that of nuclear war or even approaching it in seriousness. This is not to say, however, that there are no population problems or that what used to be called 'the population problem' has been solved. There are some striking cases of fertility reduction in Taiwan, Korea, Hong Kong and Singapore, but these affect a small proportion of the total population of the less developed countries, and the special case of China, which weighs so heavily in calculating the extent of global fertility reduction, illicitly contributes to a misleading image of continuous fertility reduction among these countries taken as a whole. In fact, the rest of the world does not display the same trend. Africa, for example, shows little fertility reduction and little interest on the part of governments. What then ought we in the US to do?

As noted before, the world is not a commons; our concern for population trends can only (and should only) be conducted through persuasion and argument with leaders of other nation-states. Since foreign population trends are threatening neither our own internal security nor the international order in a serious degree and are not likely to do so in the near future, we should display our concern through a broad appeal to principles of welfare and justice. How we should approach these issues in a particular country depends upon the nature of its society – whether it satisfies our procedural requirements mentioned earlier – and on the seriousness of the problem. Just as before, when we introduced a step ladder approach to the permissibility of interventions depending on the gravity of the problem at hand, so here a second step ladder may be introduced, this time with respect to our attitude towards other societies. First, assuming the problem is not catastrophic, we should attempt to justify to the members and leaders of the other society ethically acceptable means of arriving at government decisions while at the same time not hesitating to recommend specific means of resolving population problems. Second, if the problem is grave and direct access to the members of the society is not possible, we should at least provide our best information and policies to the dominant powers of that society. This is proper both ethically and prudentially, for it is estimated that over 90% of the net addition to the world population during the next quarter century will occur in the developing countries and the relative weight of the US and its allies will diminish radically.

In the end, painful choices will have to be made. For in the vast generality of cases that concern us in the less developed regions of the world, the values that we cherish cannot be combined easily, if at all, in population policies. This is especially so in view of the fact that it is difficult to believe that declining fertility has been due to family planning programs and so-called 'program effort'; rather, it seems that (contrary to what was inferred from the older 'Knowledge, Attitude, Practice' survey results) there was no great 'unmet demand' for contraceptives and that fertility declines began with development efforts, so that population policy must be somehow integrated into development planning as a whole. But if this point is taken seriously, as I think it should, 'population ethics' also must be integrated into the larger, disturbing, and complex field of 'development ethics'; population ethicists must turn their attention to the questions of development, its aims, definitions, and criteria, whether political, economic, psychological, or social, and the agonizing choices that attend it, especially for those sensitive to traditional values and the virtues of traditional societies.

There is, at present, no international contraceptive ethos. Should there be one? I cannot see why there should be. If anything, there must be greater understanding of the differences between the varying views and customs of different societies and peoples; indeed, I think it is a vain hope to suppose that we will be able to erect a non-trivial contraceptive ethos governing all rational people in all circumstances. The most we can hope for is a continual process of adjustment among conflicting values.

Barnard College and
Center for Population Studies,
New York

BIBLIOGRAPHY

1. Aird, J. S.: 1982, 'Population Studies and Population Policy in China', *Population and Development Review* **8**, No. 2, 267–297.
2. Bayles, M. D. (ed.): 1976, *Ethics and Population*, Schenkman Publishing Co., Cambridge, Mass.
3. Bayles, M. D.: 1980, *Morality and Population Policy*, University of Alabama Press, Ala.
4. Berelson, B. and Lieberson, J.: 1979, "Government Intervention in Fertility: What is Ethical?", *Population and Development Review* **5**, No. 4.

5. Feinberg, J.: 1974, 'The Rights of Animals and Unborn Generations', in William T. Blackstone (ed.), *Philosophy and Environmental Crisis*, University of Georgia Press, Athens, Ga.
6. Glover, J.: 1977, *Causing Death and Saving Lives*, Penguin, London, U.K.
7. Golding, M.: 1972, 'Obligations to Future Generations', *Monist* **56**.
8. Hardin, G.: 1974, 'Living on a Lifeboat', *Bioscience* **24**.
9. Hull, T. H., Hull, V. J., and Singarimbun, M.: 1977, 'Indonesia's Family Planning Story: Success and Challenge', *Population Bulletin* **32**, No. 8.
10. Isaacs, S. L.: 1981, *Population Law and Policy*, Human Sciences Press, New York, N.Y.
11. Jianguo, L. and Xiaoying, Z.: 1983, 'Infanticide in China', *New York Times*, April 11, 1983, p. 28.
12. Lieberson, J.: 1981, 'Review of Bayles, *Morality and Population Policy*', *Population and Development Review* **7**, No. 1.
13. McNicoll, G. and Nag, M.: 1982, 'Population Growth: Current Issues and Strategies', *Population and Development Review* **8**, No. 1.
14. Rawls, J.: 1971, *A Theory of Justice*, Harvard University Press, Cambridge, Mass.
15. Shue, H.: 1980, *Basic Rights*, Princeton University Press, Princeton, N.J.
16. Simon, J. L.: 1981, *The Ultimate Resource*, Princeton University Press, Princeton, N.J.
17. Veatch, R. M.: 1977, 'Governmental Population Incentives: Ethical Issues at Stake', *Studies in Family Planning* **8**, No. 4.

JANET W. SALAFF

THE RIGHT TO REPRODUCE: THE PEOPLE'S REPUBLIC OF CHINA

The idea that the [Qing] state should and did play a critical role in population growth, land use, and food supply should not come as a surprise to anyone familiar with Chinese culture and history ([66], p. 689).

[B]irth control has always been primarily an issue of politics, not of technology ([34], p. xii).

Social reproduction of the community is consequently a political endeavor, and not a natural process . . . ([78], p. 85).

Stringent restrictions on births in the People's Republic of China, without historical parallel in a civil population, have drawn a medley of reactions. This paper explores the political origins and popular responses to the recent set of state controls over family size. The question posed is: Under what circumstances can a state deny parents the right to reproduce?

Demographers refer to stringent economic and political sanctions in population control programs as 'Beyond Family Planning' measures. I will group the ethical issues raised by such programs under *economic*, *social justice* and *political* issues. Some population limitation programs appear to place the burden of a nation's *economic* advance on birth control. Critics challenge those programs that ignore the material needs of poor households that demand several able-bodied workers to maintain the household economy. This is a central issue in China.

Social justice refers to the issue of equity. Are people worse off than they otherwise would have been due to the measures? Are the same people able to benefit from improvements to their standard of living due to the measures? Or, will one set of individuals be denied its rights in exchange for an improved way of life for the future generation? To others, social justice refers to the betterment of the status of groups with a low standing. In China this particularly refers to the status of women or youth. Does the population control program improve their status, or further reduce it? [3, 29, 34].

A *political* baseline for judging programs as beyond family planning measures is whether the people view them as consistent with the

89

Stuart F. Spicker, William B. Bondeson, and M. Tristram Engelhardt, Jr.
The Contraceptive Ethos, 89–134.

mandates of the given order. Another criterion is whether measures can be maintained without undue coercion for nonconformists. Finally, measures are viewed by writers concerned with the subject of population as more acceptable if less stringent approaches have already been tried [3].

This essay first analyzes the historical background to 'Beyond Family Planning' measures in rural and urban China. It argues that the legacy of the present regime includes the protection of the peasant and working class family economy. This legacy implicates economic, social justice and political realms, and conflicts with a severe population limitation program. The paper then discusses the measures propounded in the late 1970's, and suggests that the conflict with the legacy of the family economy has forced the leaders into a stringent stance on beyond family planning policies.

PRE-1949 RURAL CHINA: BACKGROUND

Economy

In a peasant society like China, the need to reproduce the productive unit placed control over reproduction in the family, not in the hands of the individual set of parents. Reproduction was enforced by family elders and backed by community interests and pressures. Cereal, especially rice agriculture, drew mainly on family labor. Seasonal production required long-lasting cooperation to perform varied technological tasks. Families had a vested interest in remaining together to benefit from the members' combined labor, survive the nonproductive period between sowing and harvest, and prepare for the next productive period. Rice agriculture also drew together families in settled villages. Stocks, a centralized product, and a considerable infrastructure around irrigation, tools and fertilizer, demanded group, not individual, investment. The ecology promoted long-term relationships between family members and a stable family and community structure. Universal marriage, low divorce rates, high fertility and identification with the village community were the historical outcome [78, 120].

The agricultural team was often hierarchically ordered, based on gender, age, and generation. Men exerted their control over the collection and distribution of the agricultural product, although women did much farm work. Centralized management and redistribution of the product led to the election of the elder as the natural head of the family group. In China, the elder was male. Religious beliefs legitimized his role, since he managed the land on behalf of the ancestors and handed it over to future members of the family line. This productive and religious control underlay patrilineal and extended families [30, 31, 74, 109].

The cereal technology sustained only small settlements of people, from 200 in poorer villages to approximately 1000 in better-off settlements with a more diversified economic base. Many were closely related. These demographic and social constraints meant peasants sought beyond the community for young women of the proper ages to marry their sons. Exchange of wives between communities was patterned and regulated. The exchange of women enabled the elders to keep control over the women of their respective communities. Thus, along with its control over production, the family, in particular its leaders, and the community controlled the members' reproductive activities [30, 54, 111].

Before 1949, in addition to religious concerns of continuation of the ancestral line and old age support, economic structure of the family as a productive unit contributed to high levels of fertility as well. The dynamics of the life cycle gave rise to the cyclical replacement of family labor power. Parents drew on young children's labor around the home and barnyard, and in small tasks in the community like gleaning and firewood collection. But the young children were still a net loss. The peak economic needs of a household, child bearing and child rearing did not correspond with the years of highest earnings for the household unit. Mature sons and unmarried daughters, however, worked the land along with their parents; thus this life cycle stage was the most productive.

Social outlets for too few or too many offspring existed. When families could not reproduce at levels to meet their needs, minor forms of marriage and adoption prevailed. In addition, work parties and mutual aid exchanges in the community expanded adult labor power. China had a market economy. Where parents produced too many children to absorb on their small farms, they could diversify. The developed marketing system and commercial opportunities provided outlets for a labor surplus. Parents sent away their children to work and hoped eventually to receive back wages. These were means that families used to adjust their labor economic ratio in each household [16, 28, 76, 80, 81, 115, 130].

Social Justice

Families at the early stages of their cycle might have been relatively poor, but they expected to benefit when the children matured, worked side by side with the elders, and eventually replaced them in the productive economy. Thus, the key issue of distributive justice was solved when these same families that had foregone a good standard of living in the early stages, when they had many mouths to feed, could rise above subsistence in later years.

Women were disadvantaged without property rights or political power. The corporate nature of the family was derived from the jural rights of the males as basic shareholders to family property, usually land. The focus on inherited rights to ancestral property meant that control over property transmission was a central family function. Men as inheritors of property were at the core of the family. Since women had no right of ownership to the ancestral estate, they were classed as subordinates. Women's role as mothers and raisers of the valued labor force gave them a special source of influence but not power. Having children was crucial to their status in the family and community, especially the birth of sons. Women strengthened their informal status by creating networks, mainly of male progeny, upon which they could center a family that would be tied to them throughout life; this informal network has been termed the 'uterine family'. Women also contributed to the family by working in the main spheres of production. They farmed, performed wage labor, engaged in sideline activities and heavy domestic work. They socialized with neighbors and kin and kept up the personal relationships necessary for farmers' security [15, 132].

Political Issues

China was not a European-type feudal society. Landlord-peasant relations, integrated by kin ties, often took a form of patronage. The imperial system reinforced rural residence of the elite, which sustained bonds between the better-off and their home communities. For the poorest farmers, the conjugal and kinship group provided limited social services. Beyond such family-oriented services, tenants sought economic security in their relations with the wider kinship group, the clan, the village and the patron-client bond. In regions of North China, redistribution rights helped to maintain the subsistence level. Peasants could glean, obtain seeds, small agricultural tools, draught animals, dependable leases and crop reductions at times of bad harvests. Landlords' political role included that of brokers who could shield peasants from extortive state taxes and requisitions in kind, or arrange relief from the state. Landlords might provide village granaries, crop watching services, and common tenancy fields. In the best of times these exchanges protected the unproductive members of the community and the poor within the exploitive framework of the tenancy system. In Southeast China where lineages were strong, lineage leaders also buffered state-village relations, and acted as brokers for the poorer members of their lineage [30, 59, 104, 116].

From early 1800, imperial control weakened. Causes included rapid population growth that placed great pressure on natural resources. Famines and food crises occurred to an unprecedented degree and lasted through the mid-20th century. Agrarian crises made it impossible for ordinary peasants to realize the subsistence livelihood that underlay stable family life. The scarce resources were maldistributed. Political resources were strained as well. According to Jones and Kuhn, around the 1820's China's huge population required more administrative services of a scale that the Ching dynasty form of political self-regulation could not provide. Political-military organizations of the local society (secret societies and gentry militia) arose and the local elite changed its nature [45, 55, 56, 80, 124].

By the time of the Republican Revolution of 1911, the local elite bifurcated. Large landowners (the gentry elite) moved to country seats where they became urban rentiers, represented by rent collectors, with a private militia as their police force. The gentry elite no longer stood for local paternalism. Local rural headmen (in the Qing they were marginalized lower gentry, in the Republic they were often members of the local subcounty self government administration), siphoned money from villagers in league with 'local bullies.' This petty local elite and their administrative activities, usury and numerous surtaxes, impoverished local farmers, while funds never reached the central state. The military-, commerce- and government-controlled industries were other sources of elites. The world economy increasingly enmeshed villages, and world economic instability affected many poor farmers. But these elites, who did not look to the villagers to legitimate their power base, neither restored earlier forms of subsistence services, nor integrated the peasants into a new network of beneficial market exchanges [59, 116, 117, 128].

There were few outlets for the poorer tenants to obtain capital to participate in commercial agriculture and competitive cash crops in North China. Villages in Southeast and coastal China had longer experience with commercialized market activities. They came into the orbit of the cities and transferred their surplus product and people to them. Low wages and precarious employment periodically expelled workers from the capitalist sector and returned them to the rural areas. Thus workers maintained their links to the rural household to provide collective security [44, 46, 81].

Surveys in the 1930's and 1940's show a direct relationship between economic standing and household size, household complexity and surviving children. They concluded that the agrarian crisis posed a threat to the physical survival of peasant families. For example, studies of Yangtze valley, Shandong and Jiangxi province villages found that even if there was no agricultural disaster in any particular year, due to the prolonged agrarian crisis, the poor could not afford brides. Hence they were unable to reproduce to meet their economic and religious needs. The legitimacy of traditional peasant family life came into question [8, 28, 32, 33, 48, 60, 133, 160].

In many communities studied family stability and continuity were becoming a prerogative of the rich. Poor, unattached youths without land or a chance to form families were less tied to the local community. In addition to migrating for work, there is evidence that homeless villagers greatly swelled the ranks of rebel, and later communist, troops. Liberation troops in one northern village were comprised mostly of men from broken families who were unmarried and marginal because of their poverty [32, 118]. Other studies, however, believe the middle peasant formed the basis of the revolution [131]. Yet others find that rebels were tied together by the presence, not absence, of kin bonds [90]. The composition of rebel and liberation army units undoubtedly varied by area and period. But for our interest it is significant that rebel bands frequently imposed family-type and brotherhood relations on their members. This attests to the importance of a legitimate family life for the peasants which was being violated by the agrarian crisis. Further, the goals of protest often were more than banditry and violence. In one northern village, peasants joined rebel bands looking for rural self-help, self-defense, and even a restoration of patronage arrangements to help them attain the all important subsistence level [116].

Moral economists view China's 19th and 20th century rebellions as responses to the agrarian crisis, manifested as a threat to the family. This

uncertain and difficult setting of 20th century China has been character-
ized as a village society whose members took up arms to restore
traditional values of family, subsistence and security that had been
undermined. These goals were later to be honored by the political
leadership that rose to power on the wave of rural revolution. Thus,
post-1949 policies were accommodated to protect the family economy
and subsistence needs of the rural sector [32, 82, 104, 113, 117].

Economy

In urban China the economic mix changed under the Republic, when
commerce became legally secure. Recent research on modern industrial
investment in pre-war China finds a 'significant and sustained burst' of
investment activity in the small but growing modern sector ([96], p. 35).
A key feature of such investment was its regional nature. Industrial
activity focused around a small number of urban centers, notably the
Shanghai area in Southern Jiangxu province, and Manchuria, the Japanese center of investment. In China proper in 1933, the coastal area,
dominated by Shanghai, accounted for nearly two-thirds of all Chinese-
owned factories ([96], p. 30). Expansion of modern investment, production, trade and financial sectors in these regional growth centers also
stimulated the traditional economy in the centers and their hinterland.

The working-class populace maintained either a family wage or a
mixed wage and productive economy [120]. Family members pooled
their incomes and the elders exerted control over members' jobs.
Working-class families practiced a family economy because the earnings
of any one member were too low to support dependents, and women
could not support even themselves. Job insecurity and lack of pensions
further promoted the family wage economy. An authoritarian form of
childrearing contributed to parental control over children. In addition,
rural roots of the working class promoted this family form. Most male
workers in ironcasting shops and machine repair in Tianjin, and female
cotton mill workers in Shanghai, for example, were recruited from the
rural hinterland. There was also much reverse migration. Many working
adults lived as single members in the cities, and if married, their families
remained in the home village. Workers also returned to the village if
there was no work or they were needed in the harvest. Finally, small

workshops and commercial establishments run along 'traditional' paternalistic lines accounted for the majority of the urban work force, which
reinforced the family wage economy. At most, 35% of the urban work
force was found in 'modern' factories. But the social organization of
such modern factories also promoted a familistic rather than individualistic orientation [44, 46, 105, 119].

The family wage economy gave parents considerable control over
many areas of their offsprings' lives. In such a family, fertility might be
substantial because children were economically useful, and old-age
support was limited to what the family could provide [61].

For the middle classes, inheritance of property and especially family
businesses, which needed to use family labor power, contributed to a
family wage economy. However, children lost much of their economic
usefulness. Mortality levels declined, and better-off urban families had
lower infant mortality than the rest. These parents likely found it more
profitable to raise a small number of well-trained children than many
less-educated offspring. Schools also introduced new, often dissident
ideas, which reduced elite urban parents' control over their children.
The 1931 Nationalist family code, which limited the power of the family
over its members, was not applied in the countryside, but in the cities:
the code reflected and furthered family changes [60, 75, 79].

Social Justice

This new urban working class was resigned to poverty in the early years
of the family cycle. But they expected to rise above the subsistence level
later, when their children matured and went to work.

Working-class women were being drawn into urban factories; cotton
mills were the spearhead of Chinese industrialization. Yet working-class
women did not use their new economic opportunities to fight for
freedom from the family. They were more likely to use their economic
status to improve the family in which they grew up, and into which they
married [61, 119].

Elite youths, to the contrary, began to rebel against tight control of
their elders early in the century. They had access to the new, often
dissident, ideas from outside and within China, and expressed their
resistence to family controls over marriage, for example. Feminist ideas
flourished among these families, as reflected in the May 4th movement
of 1919, which was in good part a youth rebellion [75, 79, 113].

Political Issues

The Japanese occupation greatly affected the coastal centres. In Tsinan and Tianjin, industry stagnated, expanded slightly, then declined with the decline of the economy after the start of the Pacific war. Urban poverty, exacerbated by wartime dislocations and inflation, threatened the ability of workers to maintain their families. The urban working class sought a stable and strong family life [7, 44].

The urban elite perceived the economic, political and cultural turbulence of the twentieth century as a crisis to the patriarchy. The 'family revolution' espoused by the children of the intellectual elite attacked parental control. Goals were: the elimination of the double sexual and economic standard and of multiple 'wives', and freedom of marriage and divorce. These goals found their way into the early platform of the communist movement in the 1920's. But they were later downplayed or removed altogether in favor of issues relevant to the rural populace and working class that demanded a stronger family life [48, 113].

Thus, for the urban populace, some 15% of China's population, the family system was also in decline. But concerns varied by social class. The working class felt the basis of its family economy threatened, and wanted to strengthen it, while the elite attacked parental control over family members. The views of both sectors of urbanites focused on family reform. But only one group – the urban elite youths – sought freedom of the individual from the family. The remainder sought a stronger family with the right to survive, marry and reproduce in numbers that would strengthen their family economy [113].

AFTER THE REVOLUTION: 1949 THROUGH THE 1970'S IN RURAL CHINA

Economy

Land reform in the 1950's undermined the power of wealthy elite families. The integration of rural productive units into the collectively managed economy, completed in the first decade of communist power, further shifted the power of the community to the non-elite. The non-elite was defined at the time of land reform as the nonexploiter of labor, the poor and lower-middle peasant family. Nevertheless, "peasant patriarchy was not destroyed; it was further democratized and secured" ([113], p. 204).

The 'new socialist patriarchy', a term coined by Stacey, derived firstly from political strictures against geographical and social mobility. A peasant inherited his occupational status from birth, from the mother's peasant standing. Political status was derived from the father's class status, which was established in the father's line at the time of rural social class classification, usually as land reform. Membership in a production team or village was also derived from the father's local place. Mobility was limited, with few channels available for exiting from the rural area [93, 113].

Labor-intensive farming methods of production also continued family control over its members [113]. The development of Chinese agriculture, despite considerable modern inputs and institutional reforms, rarely took the form of 'factories in the fields' envisioned by the 1958 Great Leap Forward. That is, there was not an assembly line division of labor with wages or pensions accruing to the individuals [92]. Until 1980, production teams organized labor input. Some writers argue that the production team drew its members from Chinese lineage segments and therefore resembled a kinship unit [65]. Others find that the teams were deliberately structured to draw on members of varied lineage segments [93]. Nevertheless, team members often had some kin ties with each other.

The household head still provided a workforce for the team, and mobilized family labor power for the team economy. To maintain output, the collective allied with the family and its personal ties that got production out. This continued peasant family control over labor power, or a family productive economy [17, 113].

The livelihood of the peasant household was shaped directly by the local economy. Until 1980, rural productive units distributed collective income in cash and kind. The amount each family gained was linked to the profitability and productivity of the products, after an amount for tax, reinvestment and social services was retained by the collective. The distributed collective income was based on each person's subsistence needs and on 'work points' earned by those participating in collective labor. The work point system abided by the rule "from each according to his ability, to each according to his labor". However, "A work point . . . sets a value on a given work form in relation to all other forms of work performed by team members. The value of a work point is not an absolute value but a value in proportion. . . . In a team that is doing well, the value of a work point will be higher" ([93], p. 470). In many areas diversification of the local economy proceeded to expand income beyond that obtainable from agriculture. Small-scale industries based on local raw materials (bricks and hand fans), put out on contract from cities (sewing garments), or contracted labor to cities (construction), increased collective income. Remuneration to the collective (not the individual worker) enlarged the total sum of product, the base for calculating work points [24, 85, 93].

Despite industrial inputs, therefore, the rural productive economy (until 1980) tied peasants' rewards closely to the fate of the collective. Solidarity persisted between households to get out production. The exchange of goods and services was institutionalized in the coincidence of production and residence. Villagers engaged in "an unprecedented level of exchange of goods and services" ([17], p. 179). Few avenues of escape from the pressures of primary groups existed. Consequently, through various sanctions at their disposal, the older generation maintained control over the norms of the local community, which enabled it to modify the new ideology in its own interests. The concentration and overlapping of primary groups for production, consumption and welfare reinforced parental control over family formation [87].

Within the household, the principal divisions of labor were still sexual and generational. The patrilocal household remained the norm. The family productive economy demanded the efforts of all members to survive and prosper. Women averaged lower wages than men. They performed different tasks, and these were rated as less valuable than those of men. But women still contributed their labor to the major sectors of the economy. These included the income-earning contribution from the collective sector, sideline activities of the private sector, and the non-economic earning contribution within the domestic sphere [1, 17, 23, 54, 87, 113].

Children still needed to earn their keep. Peasants raised livestock privately for consumption and sale and engaged in other cottage industries. In one village in the mid-1960's in Guangdong province, children earned half an adult's income minding pigs and geese. Need for their income deterred parents from sending children to primary school: one-quarter of the province's rural children did not attend school. Girls had the least opportunity. In one extreme case in 1970, only two of the 40 village primary school pupils were girls ([122], pp. 53–55, 265).

Rural poverty required that people form families. Lardy has argued that the state used its centralized system of planning to achieve a better

distribution of income between rural and urban areas, and between
more and less productive regions ([63], pp. 159, 192). It has also been
estimated that per capita income doubled between 1952 and 1957 [63].
Nevertheless, from the 1950's through the 1970's, the state had to keep
farm product purchase prices low and drew surplus from rural areas to
invest in industry. The average income of the rural populace barely rose
between 1957 and 1977 ([63], p. 22). There was no comprehensive
welfare system, and it fell to each family to support its unproductive
members [6, 20, 21]. Under such circumstances, the populace protected
its right to form families, and to form large ones.

Social Justice

Within the collective, the ratio of earnings between the top and bottom
quintiles ranged from 2:1 to 3:1. The higher earners were in an advanced stage in their family cycle, with many adult earners and few
non-earners. Since individual skill and physical strength determined
earnings, the dependency ratio and number of able-bodied workers set
the family income level. A family with many children and few adult
earners, as in the past, suffered from a low living standard in the short
run. But such a family's earning power was cyclical. It bore children 'for
the future' [6, 58] ([83], p. 35) [103, 123].

In contrast to the pre-1949 period, however, some local collectives
tried to help those families in poverty who had many dependent offspring to support. One method of help by the rural unit that was used
during periods of intense egalitarianism (1958–1959 and 1966–1973) was
to readjust the labor point system. Since a large proportion of collective
income was distributed to members according to their work perform-
ance, inequality was reduced by raising that share of all income distributed according to need. In addition, during the Cultural Revolution,
the system of work points was altered to reward those with good
attitudes, but only unskilled and poorly remunerated work perform-
ance. Within such collectives, "the redistribution effects are particularly
significant . . . where production is relatively low and food consumption
accounts for a large share of total family expenditure" ([85], pp. 58–59).

In the process of aiding the family economy of those with weak
demographic structures, the state underwrote high fertility. For example, a village in Fujian province alleviated the poverty of families with
many small children by allowing them an overdraft on their incomes
from the collective economy. These were like interest-free loans, which

allowed the villagers to defer payment until their children could work on the team, thus paying off the cost of their own upbringing. Counties also sold extra rice to poor brigades with many low-income families. There was also an incentive to have children in a time of grain shortage. Villagers calculated that the grain ration allotted each child was more than adequate for its needs, leaving a small surplus for adult consumption. In addition, each child was given a plot of land and other rations. Families with few children generally had to purchase high-priced rice on the black market when their rations ran short. But families with many children often sold rice in order to raise additional cash. "Villagers felt it was better to have children than to have to purchase rice on the black market, because in the end . . . [they had] something to show for it" ([70], p. 8) ([83], p. 35).

The rural economy that was based on strong households and family units placed women in dependent positions. The family was still patri-local and village exogamous in most areas, which gave women little power or influence outside their home. A study of the implementation of the marriage law of 1950 argued that by the mid-1950's the leaders dropped the 'radical phase' in order to protect the peasant household economy. Although women held legal right to land, without state backing they were unable to remove their land from the household to manage it by themselves [54]. Due to village exogamy, women who were married did not contribute to their natal households, and parents were reluctant to spend money and time educating their daughters for non-traditional roles [23]. One comprehensive study found that despite collectivization, women remained tied to traditional roles. No more than 20 to 30% of the work force of commune and brigade enterprises were comprised of women in 1975; the same was true in 1980 ([1], pp. 167, 173) [18]. Given this dependence on the patriarchal unit, there was still reason for women to bear sons to obtain influence through their biological family.

Parents could still control or influence their offsprings' marriage choices, since the younger generation had little individual economic choice outside the village in which it grew up. 'Free choice' marriage appeared to be relatively rare. Where old guidelines to marriage were broken down, cadres helped youths find mates [17, 87, 101]. Thus, there was no place for the unmarried, and a 0.1% sample survey in 1982 found the percentage of women who remained single all their lives was small, with most marrying before they reached age 35. Marital relations

were stable. Women who had been divorced or remarried only accounted for 4.49% of the total number of married women of childbearing age [136]. The choice of a mate, or even family size was made on the
basis of family needs. These needs were pronatalist.

Political Issues

The political basis of the revolution in the rural areas shaped the
leadership's commitment to the survival and subsistence economy of the
peasant household. The need to get out rural production and to maintain political legitimacy led to this outcome. Thus for the first time in
historical memory, peasants were assured their economic and social
continuity. This rested on their having a household with enough strong
workers for family subsistence, and even the chance for prosperity.
Parental control over the fruits of the family members' labor underlay
control over other areas of family life, and limited the rebellion of youth
and women. Such control also had pronatalist implications, since parents believed that if they bore many children, they could count on the
children to help the household economy.

The Chinese leadership, however, was aware of the need to limit
population growth, and unfolded birth control campaigns in the countryside in the early 1970's [13, 89, 102]. Why did these not take root? For
one reason, local leaders were under pressure to support poor households in their collectives. Decentralization of economic resources also
gave them some powers to resist the center. Nevertheless, and overriding this, power still flowed from the centralized state structure [9]. Thus,
Lardy argues that the state retained "substantial power to determine the
expenditure of local governments" ([63], p. 135). Membership in the
communist party and submission to brigade and commune authorities in
many productive spheres meant village leaders were accountable to the
state. Mass campaigns to limit rural fertility failed because of the
sanctions built into the organization of local production and services
that supported substantial fertility.

Thus in some areas parents limited their family size only when they
were already aged 30 to 35 and presumably had several children [100].
In other areas, fertility remained "uncontrolled" [70]. We know now
from the .1% sample survey of 1982 that the average number of children
borne by women of childbearing age (total fertility rate) rose from 5.4 in
the 1940's to 5.6 in the 1950's, to 5.7 in the 1960's, before dropping to
4.0 in the 1970's [94]. Since the poverty of families with small children

was often reduced by local arrangement, families themselves suffered less in the short run from their excess fertility and gained when children matured.

Economy

The conditions for the family wage economy attenuated. Parental control over household members was loosened, if not broken. Crucial to this was the introduction of public, largely state-paid education, "and the accompaniment of the parent by the state as partner in the selection of adult work roles for the maturing person" ([95], p. 175). Careers for youths depended partly on their level of education and the specialty of the high school they attended. Educational opportunities were concentrated in the cities. The Chinese school system was based on the 12-year American model. By the mid-1960's nearly all children attended primary school, and most primary school graduates expected to enter junior high school, which was academic based. Senior high school provided academic preparation for attending a university and accommodated a fraction of the junior high school students. Only a proportion of senior high school graduates entered universities, while the rest entered the work force, or, as jobs became difficult to find in the mid-1960's, went to the countryside or remained without work. The majority of junior high school graduates went to work directly from school. Others opted for vocational schooling that provided terminal training for specific white collar or blue collar careers [122].

Access to schools depended partly on children's achievement on examinations and partly on the political heritage of social class designation from birth. The mix of these factors varied by the political period: academic qualifications weighed relatively heavily during the First Five Year Plan, and again from 1961 to 1963; at other times the 'class line' outweighed academic achievement [122].

Parents were able to influence their children's achievement level in accordance with their class-based resources. The former middle classes and professionals had above average education, while workers were usually semi-literate. The better educated could help their children in school work directly, or indirectly provide role models or encouragement for higher expectations. If parental social networks linked into higher-level bureaucratic jobs, children also attempted higher levels of education to prepare themselves for such jobs. Consequently, their children outnumbered and outperformed children of workers in the 'keypoint' (model) schools and academic high schools, according to one study of Guangdong schools ([122], pp. 26–27). Costs were another factor. They flowed partly from tuition and supplies, which, while not very high, amounted to around 6% of a worker's monthly income ([122], p. 21). Paying the fees for several children was burdensome, and a keypoint school with dormitory and meals was even more costly. Parents also had to do without the earnings of young adolescent children for longer periods if the children attended high school or specialized vocational school.

Until 1965, students upon graduation from junior high had a variety of options open to them, with only those determined to seek university entrance moving on to a regular senior high. Nationally only 9% of all secondary school students were enrolled in regular senior high schools. However, there was great urban variation, with nearly half of Shanghai secondary school students in regular high schools. Parents set their goal for their children's education on an assessment of the likelihood of the children continuing along the academic ladder and the jobs they might get from attending different levels and types of schools. Aspirations varied by the parents' class background. Working-class parents aimed for blue-collar jobs for their children, available through junior high school certification. The more ambitious sought a specialty (e.g., accounting) through vocational high school. Children of the former middle classes, intellectuals and revolutionary cadres aimed for academic high school and college, despite the small proportions accepted into regular high school (360,000 students in 1976), and the difficulties for those graduates who did not enter college (in 1976, 54%) in getting jobs ([98], p. 7) ([122]; pp. 47–48).

Virtually all schools closed during the Cultural Revolution in 1966, and opened two years later on an experimental basis. Promotion from junior to a shortened senior high school was common, and focused on regular high schools, which increased in number to accommodate the crowds. Currently, however, senior high school accepts few junior high school graduates, and academic competition has reemerged ([98], p. 7) ([122], pp. 207–217).

The educational competition, most intense for the parents that harbored higher academic and job aspirations for their children, affected family size goals. Urban fertility, in contrast to the pre-1949 period, was probably indirectly related to social standing. Former middle-class parents and intellectuals felt that they could devote themselves to preparing their children for school promotion if they bore fewer children. In addition to competitive educational goals, after collectivization of industry was completed by the mid-1950's, private capital could not be reinvested for personal profit. Family firms were eliminated, and family income derived from wages earned outside the home. Wages of the former middle strata, intellectuals and revolutionary cadres were high enough so that they did not need numerous children to support a household economy. Middle-strata wives who held elite women's jobs that demanded higher education were reluctant to spend much time in caring and rearing several youngsters. Finally, the recent widening of opportunities to buy consumer goods at high cost competed with the desire for a number of children ([87], p. 44) [100].

Working-class parents were likely to have higher fertility since their living situations differed. Their choice of a lower terminal school year reduced the direct costs of offspring [122]. While parents could no longer send children to earn a living before age 16, pooling of household earnings still existed [21]. Parents counted on their sons to contribute their wages when they entered the labor force. The key question was therefore whether working-class parents would bear numerous children to expand the family rice pot.

The answer appeared to depend on the nature of the parent's working-class jobs, which differed greatly by the ownership and size of the unit. State sector factory jobs were secure, promoted by seniority and gave high wages. These wages were regulated by grades which were set by the state, not the particular unit. While urban wages remained unchanged for two decades after 1957, and in real terms may have dropped as much as 20%, nevertheless, the income may have been adequate for parents to survive without depending on their grown children's input. Security, which was crucial to the working class, reduced one source of high fertility for these state sector workers. The enterprise met a wide range of economic and social needs. Units widely accepted the recommendations of their work force for new employees and frequently took on workers' children. Job security and the recommendation system was referred to as the 'iron rice bowl'. State sector factories provided solid retirement pensions, which were adequate for elderly workers to live on. Moreover, upon their retirement, workers had the right to pass a job in their units to one child. State sector units, which comprised 83% of the male labor force in 1982, varied, however, by the size of the unit. The larger units had more resources and could provide housing and even hospitals to their work force. Smaller units and county-level factories may have lacked these social perquisites. The wide ranging features of the large state sector factory jobs brought the workers into close identification with their units. In addition, the presence of the party and activist members fostered social control. These features may have been absent in smaller state sector units. Nevertheless, state sector workers' solid economic situation allowed them to survive on their own wages [110, 114, 125].

Minor pronatalist elements existed in these perquisites through the mid-1970's. The municipality or work unit allocated housing by demand, and large families got priority. Further, staff and workers with many children, who could not support them on their salaries, obtained subsidies. (Nevertheless, a study of people on welfare in other nations concluded that it is unlikely that parents bear many children on purpose in order to obtain more state aid [135].)

More research is needed on workers in large and small collective factories and neighborhood enterprises. In 1981 these collective sector workers comprised 23% of the non-agricultural labor force. Wages averaged 79% of the wages of state unit workers, pensions were lower, and collectives met fewer of the workers' needs ([114], p. 433). Did these workers require more children to fill up the family rice pot?

Where family income was low, the number of employed family members compensated for low income. In fact a survey of 46 cities and towns in 1981 found that average per capita income of families varied directly with the number of employed members. Size of earnings was much less important than number of workers in setting the per capita income in the household ([114], p. 438). On the other hand, collective units varied by their size, and better wages and conditions were found in those units attached to state sector factories. Moreover, only 17% of the male labor force were in the collective sector. Thus, women were disproportionately represented in the collective economy: in 1981 women constituted 36% of the labor force and 50.6% of the collective labor force [114]. Because women lacked pensions, they, along with women that did not perform wage work, had to look to their children to support them in their old age ([18], p. 122). Nevertheless, since few women remained unmarried, their income, however low, was added to their husbands'. The combined income of both parents was superior to the low average wage implied by figures on the collective sector. Thus, this sector of urbanites may also have had enough to live and retire on without demanding the input of several strapping children.

Finally, the urban division of labor and dispersal of primary groups weakened kin and family head control over their offspring. Cities were organized into neighborhoods, which were subdivided into residential groups of from 150 to 500 households. Their main activities included the establishment of kindergartens, community service stations and small-scale neighborhood factories; they conducted political campaigns among residents. Urban neighborhoods organized the unemployed community members, while workers organized at their production locales. Husband and wife were often separately organized. As a result, urban neighborhoods did not constitute unified production, distribution and accounting units typical of rural neighborhoods.

The dispersal of primary groups in cities provided a wide range of connections to reference groups and options. Most urbanites came into contact with a variety of behavioral patterns. Young people were likely to take the advice of or follow examples of peers, members of their school, work units or political associations [95, 122].

Urban parents looked to strong ties, like kin, more distant circles, like former classmates or more indirect ties ('gwanxi') to obtain assistance. But these ties did not make parents closely dependent on their kin. Dependence on interpersonal ties covered fewer of urbanites' daily needs than of people in the rural sector, for in this period peasants depended on local ties to get production out. Moreover, those whom the urbanites looked to for assistance did not themselves form a dense group, in which everyone knew each other and held common values. Hence, even if urban kin pressed for many offspring, pressures were not organized so effectively as to override the limitations of urban material life [17].

Social Justice

The question of whether working class parents had to maintain a family wage economy in which all earners contributed to the household budget bears on the issue of social justice. If the older folk could not survive without numerous offspring, and if their own children in turn expected the same fate, then they found stringent family size limits unjust. If, on the contrary, there was financial flexibility, and the household head could do without the earnings of grown children and even contribute to

their support (if they were without work or were sent to the countryside), such a household economy was not pronatalist. The working class
did not need to bear many children to survive in later years, and relaxed
its hold over its offspring as a result. From the material at hand, it is
likely that the family wage economy was crucial mainly for the minority
of male collective sector workers, while the rest might have wished for
more children but did without.

Relatively disadvantaged urbanites included women. Women held
jobs in a range of types of units. Andors' comprehensive study concludes that the most disadvantaged women were those that worked in
neighborhood service stations or collective workshops. These women
were the relatively poorly educated, with ordinary factory jobs that they
quit upon bearing several children. They worked in small units that
offered few alternatives to a 'familist' orientation. On the other hand,
these women worked outside the home. There they interacted with
women who were not their kin, which might have mitigated the prona-
talism of an environment with low ceilings on pay and opportunities
([1], pp. 118–119). In contrast, women in state units, where child care
facilities existed and pay was higher, remained there throughout their
family building. They seemed more open to identification with their
units, and less to traditional family roles.

Unemployed youths deserve our attention, for they comprised the
bulk of the unemployed (who were an estimated nine to 18% of the
urban labor force). More than two-thirds were women ([127], pp. 2–4).
In China it was hard for men to marry without a job, rations or a place
to live. Thus, young men without work were not likely to swell the ranks
of early parents, although they did so in other third-world settings.

Political Issues

Except in muted terms, with reference to collective interest, urbanites
no longer advocated the May 4, 1919 slogans of equality of the individual against family control, freedom of divorce, and of women [113].
Nevertheless, the urban occupational structure, with its minutely strat-
ified grades and hierarchies of wages and conditions that covered most
workers, encouraged competition over distribution of status and material goods. Parents competed with neighbors and colleagues, and within
their occupation and between occupations to improve their living standard within the regime's tolerated limits. This led to a form of individual
pursuit of interests. Thus, an uneasy balance was forged between the

goal of a collective orientation and pursuit of material interests. Indeed, the journal *Red Flag* chastised urban couples who thought that "marriage is only a personal affair". It stressed that while the family in the present society was basically different from that in the old (pre-1949) society, "it is still the cell of our society and as the basic unit of people's lives, the family still shoulders various social responsibilities" [127]. Urban couples went too far in the direction of individual pursuit of their small family interests.

Within the family, youths also pursued their separate interests, especially youths who had post-primary and post-junior high school education. David Raddock has shown the powerful magnet that the school and peer group had on the attitudes and behaviors of adolescents. He finds that the formal institutions and informal peer groups often drew youths into open or suppressed conflict with their parents. Within this group of better educated youths, mainly from politically disfavored backgrounds, parents will no longer reward their children for close adherence to the family. Many could not depend on their children for support either. Parents appeared to have responded to the immense urban changes by becoming more democratic in their childrearing. Raddock documents the emergence of 'horizontal' father-son relationships where fathers liberally encouraged their sons to seek peers and pursue important goals outside the family. Such parents thus fostered in their sons greater independence than was true in the past [95].

In sum, by the 1970's, many or most urban couples were able to think of their family size goals in terms of a household with input from fewer members. Although they may have borne sizable families, they were prepared to reduce family size in the future without great difficulty. The units in the cities promoted antinatalist campaigns for many years. However, parents were likely to focus mainly on the material requirements of their household rather than the units' demands in setting their family size [100].

COLLECTIVE CONTROL OVER CHILDBEARING: LATE 1970's–1983: RURAL CHINA

Economy

In the post-Mao era, China's modernization goals depend closely on further raising levels of production and reducing population growth rates. Both require substantial organizational change. China was able to sustain a relatively rapid rate in growth of the domestic product of 6% since 1952 ([63], p. 192). But it is estimated that both agricultural productivity and population growth averaged two to three percent per year during the same period ([12], p. 20). Agriculture has thus barely kept up with population growth. The new policies 'attack' both sides of the production/population equation ([113], p. 269). They seek to raise agricultural growth to over 4% and lower population growth to one percent each year.

The leadership uses systems analysis to arrive at the average birth rate needed to reach the desired population size. Some scholars posit an optimal target of 0.7 billion people, which requires a reduction in the total population which was 1.03 billion in 1982. If a one-child family is adopted universally, the population size will peak in the year 2000 and decline thereafter to 700 million in the year 2040. Others aim for a decline of 1.2 million in the year 2000. If the populace bears an average of one and one-half children, this goal can be reached.

Other estimates give the social costs of raising a child to age 16, including education: rural areas, 1600 yuan; rural townships, 4800 yuan; cities, 6900. They also assess the extent to which population growth offsets economic productivity. If the population remains stable, gross national product (GNP) will show a yearly increase of 6.8%, enabling a per capita income of $1,000 (US) by the year 2000. But if every woman of childbearing age gives birth to an average of two children, a yearly increase in GNP of 8.1% will be needed to reach the same per capita figure. These and other calculations inform the population policy today ([10], p. 68) [39, 40, 47, 71, 112, 138, 143].

In order to raise production levels in rural areas, the leadership has restored public legitimacy to the private sector. Households can now subcontract the cultivation of the production team's collective land. Peasant families are granted loans and access to fodder lands to encourage private livestock raising and sideline production [11].

The logic of the rural household economy has maintained high fertility. Collectivization and social policy has eased the burden of additional dependents for the family. The new encouragement to family production in the collective still appears to demand several strapping, hardworking offspring. Even the new marriage law (adopted in 1980), which requires children to support their parents, confirms offspring centrality in the social welfare system [113]. This production system which fosters the family's role as a unit of labor and profit is proving a major stumbling block to lowering family size to a single child.

Whereas the material incentives expand the area of private initiative, the opposite is the case with population policy [14, 113]. Articles 2 and 12 of the new marriage law and Article 53 of the new 1978 Constitution enjoin the couple to practice family planning. Indeed, family planning may be the chief force behind revising the marriage law. There have been major organizational changes to reconcile production incentives with the needed low population growth rate. These have severed the right to reproduce from parents and their kin, and have placed this right firmly in the hands of the collective political units.

How is the leadership able to enforce its decisions? The term 'organizational competence' refers to the meshing of structures that permit leaders to assess and act on an overly-high demographic growth rate. Through the 1970's the rural organizational leadership manifested such competence because administrative–political units dominated operational units. The rural collective always assumed ultimate responsibility to deploy labor and disburse income while leaving the production and mobilization of labor power to families. Dependent children reduce the sum of capital that could be directed to retained savings for the purpose of mechanizing production, or to the infrastructure. Because of the high birth rate, teams and brigades diverted their profits to pay for maternity leave and village schools. Commune leaders were thus able to assess the costs to their own resources of the high population growth rates of the units under them [68, 77, 121].

Higher-level units, at the county, province and above, also suffer from the burden of a dependent populace with a large proportion of nonproductive children. If an area is not well off, brigades may purchase grain from the county. Further, Lardy points out that although many Western visitors have the impression that the system of communal health care is self financed, the state underwrites a "very large portion of rural health expenditures". Some provinces report that 70 to 80% of all budgetary funds expanded for health are allocated to rural areas, indicating the importance of the county-level budget in the delivery of medical care in rural areas. (The county budget remains an integral component of the unified national budget). The health system provides the basic family planning services, and brigade clinics and commune hospitals are funded from retained funds with county subsidies. The higher the brigade's productive level, the more funds are invested in the medical care system. Thus, one can surmise that local public health personnel do not profit from a high birth rate and more babies. Thus, once family size limitation has been defined as a priority for collective action, health personnel are easily included in the network that motivates parents to limit their family size. In addition, teachers in rural primary schools are also often paid through the county budget ([63], p. 167). Since counties subsidize services for many poorer brigades, the costs of a rapidly growing population are felt at each administrative/ productive level.

The local statistical system is being brought into the population control picture. A new hierarchy of reporting vital statistics upwards from a local Birth Planning Cadre parallels the long standing, less detailed household registration system. According to one observer, when these statistics are combined with information from the team accountant on labor power, a relatively accurate picture of the population size changes emerges [64]. However, another visitor to several rural areas finds that the birth statistics are underreported and do not tally with the population statistics of recent years. He believes this is due less to a concern to keep births low for political reasons, and more to a lack of interest in statistical accuracy ([4], pp. 127–129). Nevertheless, it is clear that the local statistical system is used to reinforce population control efforts.

When in the 1970's demographic growth threatened social stability and economic advance, this hierarchical yet decentralized administrative structure helped leaders define and act on the situation. Local costs of high fertility coincided with the felt costs to the county and with national attention to the slowing population growth. The collective leadership then began to integrate family reproductive plans congruently into its economic plans.

For example, the leadership in the 'model' county of Shifang, Sichuan, (a model unit is held up for emulation by other units), evaluated the ratio of arable land per capita and per laborer, and the proportions of land devoted to basic grains versus other cash crops. They found that the stress on basic grain crops of the cultural revolution era made it hard to divert land to the more profitable cash crops (in this case, tobacco). Even worse, due to high population growth the amount of land tilled per laborer decreased in the 1960's despite more arable land having been brought under cultivation [70].

Local leaders redressed the situation by withdrawing from households the right to determine family size. They promoted the two-child family as the rural maximum, and the one-child family as the ideal. To enforce these stringent norms the state tried to bring administrative, political and production units into line. The balance of the new incentives will now favor small family norms.

Production units have ended collective supports to large families, where they existed. Interest-free loans and extra grain rations are no longer forthcoming for large families. Instead, there are new economic supports for small families. These vary by the productivity of the area. In Shifang county, Sichuan, before the dismantling of the collective economy, in a single-child household, the child obtains (1) one and one-half private plots of land (these are normally small, but provide much of a family's cash); (2) one basic adult ration from birth (normally a three-year old child obtains 40% of the adult ration; a seven-year old obtains 80%; (3) subsidized medical health care fees; (4) free cooperative medical subscription and free admission to the pre-primary and primary school system; and (5) priority in applications in the future for change of residence, jobs, admissions to school and welfare assistance. Parents obtain: (1) the promise of post-retirement and insurance support based on their previous workpoint earning levels; (2) work opportunities for those still capable of working at retirement time; (3) well administered village homes for the elderly without kin [70].

These awards are revoked if a second child is born. But if more than two children, or too closely spaced children are born, parents are actually penalized. Violators of the small family norm: (1) will be docked ·10% of their work points; (2) will obtain no paid maternity leave; (3) will pay their own medical expenses for pregnancy and delivery; and (4) will pay for the child's nursery, kindergarten, and school tuition [70].

In 1979, a Fujian village promoted the two-child family, with four years between births. To attain this goal it imposed the following restrictions: After the birth of her first child the mother was required to agree to an IUD insertion at the commune hospital before she could register the baby's birth; The family obtained its allotted grain ration, free plot and other rations for the new member only upon registration; After five years the couple could apply to the commune for permission to have the IUD removed for a second pregnacy; After the second birth, the husband or wife was required to agree to sterilization, or enter a contract that stipulated that if they chose another form of birth control, an accidental pregnancy would be aborted. Failure to comply meant this child would not be registered. Couples that agreed to sterilization after the birth of their first child were given in lump sum a sewing machine, 30 yuan and 50 catties of rice [83].

It is clear that these new economic sanctions behind the small family can only be meaningful in a poor country. Basic necessities such as food or rations are stressed. It is also clear that many of these perks such as old age homes have not been widely available [22].

Economic payments must be sizable to make a difference to families in order to convince farmers that prosperity does not turn on having a strong family structure. Cadres in Dayi country, Sichuan, argued to the populace that a child that qualified for the one-child certificate would earn, on the basis of current earnings, between 1500 and 1600 yuan by the age of 14 from the various awards; this was 'no small sum' it was pointed out. Furthermore, they stated, children did not always care for their old parents: "When small, children are little darlings, but when they marry, they leave home. When there is no money, the babies are looked after first and then the old folks". The solution was to develop the economy: "In some production teams where [annual] income averages more than 250 yuan, the income of peasants being almost that of urban workers, the income and life being rather prosperous, old folks have little to worry about" [70]. This argument can hardly convince peasants since urban workers actually earn over 50 yuan per month, plus bonuses and perquisites [114].

Further, the new rural production responsibility system encourages peasants to think directly of their family strength as a key to their livelihood. The production responsibility system links work performed with remuneration received. As practiced in a commune in Hubei, the land is distributed according to a formula that is fixed on the number of standard male laborers a household has ([11], p. 19). It thus shows that households have claim to more land and higher earnings if they have a strong family structure [129]. Further, families that meet and surpass their production quotas can in many areas sell their surplus and earn funds that are not controlled by the collective. As a result, peasants are reported to believe they now can manage to make ends meet despite having many children. At any rate, they are prepared to take the consequences of their poverty. "We farm our own land; we eat our own grain; and when we have a lot of children, we raise them ourselves" [26].

The new economic system makes it difficult for the leadership to enforce a small child family norm. The amount a peasant couple receives in exchange for reducing its size becomes a crucial bargaining lever. But, as more productive land and resources are withdrawn from the collective by families on a contract basis, it becomes that much more difficult for collectives to obtain the funds to pay peasants for small families. At the same time, cadres lose the power to enforce compliance to the directives over peasants who are no longer directly under their economic leadership [19, 107, 139].

Cadres themselves are pressed to take the population movement as seriously as they treat movements for raising production output. The press criticizes cadres for slackening their leadership or adopting a laissez-faire attitude toward birth control. It is clear from the press that the campaign for a one-child family is difficult to enforce among leaders and parents [67].

To overcome these problems, a system of fines or taxes has been suggested by which peasants on contract will pay for their disobedience to the small child family norms. Those families that comply will receive the funds in turn. Other areas give bonuses to families that meet production and birth quotas [84, 141, 143]. Production units report mixed reactions. Some wealthy areas, such as suburban collectives that can afford old age homes and even pensions, retain sufficient resources to continue these rewards under the production responsibility system. Their families appear to comply. Other productive units are less well situated and have fewer collective resources. Their families feel that by going it alone they will become most prosperous, and that a large family is the key to success. Leaders emphasize to the peasants that low productivity can only be solved in the long run by increased mechanization, which can only come from savings which the growth rate imperils [39, 57, 71, 134]. One can further envision a return to mutual aid forms of labor exchanges, which were common in the past when families lacked sufficient labor power of their own to till their land or harvest crops. One such multi-household labor organization was in fact formed in a brigade in Guizhou in order to pool lands and labor power ([11], p. 31).

The right to set one's family size thus shifted from the family and kin groups to the collective and its political leadership. Initially, this stringent program did not place the entire burden of economic advance upon limiting births or upon the birth control of the poor. A systematic program of extraction and redistribution of capital investment through material inputs was expected to coincide with the birth control program. Indeed, local units defended the policy to their members on the basis of the increased capital they could accumulate with a smaller population. Nevertheless, the production responsibility system has acknowledged limitations in the area of collective accumulation and deployment of resources. The system impedes brigade industries, scientific experiments, use of large farm machinery, and planning and implementing basic construction ([11], pp. 29–30). These limitations place questions on the ability of the collective to give a proper economic exchange for families' acquiescence of their birth rights.

Social Justice

The leadership is trying to forge a link between the economic fate of the family and the collective or nation in the short and long terms. In addition to altering the incentive system, the party and mass organizations use political means to encourage the peasants to think less in terms of their own household economy and more in terms of the future of the nation. Cadres visit each couple individually, meet with kin that object to a couple's limiting births, and hold mandatory study sessions on population policy. These sessions are called 'drawing up accounts.' Counties draw up and publish accounts of the population, arable land and food grain in their areas; communes, brigades and teams follow suit. The accounts consist of: the period after liberation, the current period and that of the year 2000. The purpose of keeping accounts is to show the dire straits of the land/population ratio due to past high fertility, and to offer two scenarios for the future: less land if population is not controlled well, and an 'excellent situation' in each local area if family planning is earnestly carried out [139].

Parents thus learn to link their personal fates with that of the collective. Cadres are urged to explain to commune members that each individual is both a producer and consumer of wealth. When a farm household has a newborn child, it must be fed, clothed, housed and educated before it is old enough to work. This entails costs. When this message is properly conveyed, peasants understand the difficulties confronting the state and learn that uncontrolled population growth bears heavily on their own family economy [67].

Meetings take several forms. Heiliongjiang brigades reported having greatly lowered population growth by holding meetings of mothers- and daughters-in-law, and of unmarried youths, "to let the masses use their personal knowledge and experience to enlighten each other". Meetings are also conducted at which cadres urge participants to make collective decisions about allocating births to members [14, 43, 64].

The state issues quotas to give birth, which units allocate to members. By all accounts these are issued equitably, based on demographic characteristics. 'Birth rights' are allocated to families on the basis of the slogan, 'Late, spaced, few'. Priority to give birth in some areas goes to childless married couples, next to couples with one older child, and finally to couples whose single child was born more recently. In other areas, any couple that is married may have the first child [107]. Charts that record the reproductive histories of local women and their planned reproduction schedule are posted. The charts publicize the numbers and ages of children, each couple's chosen method of birth control, and the year in which they have been authorized to have a child, if any ([14, 64]).

But the family basis of the household economy remains crucial. Numerous surveys have been conducted on the desired family size of the populace. In rural areas, no more than 5% of the subjects prefer one child and over two-fifths wish for three or more. A report on Dayi county, Sichuan province, describes the results of their survey: only 20% of the peasants fully support the new single-child family norm, and 15% actively oppose it. They claim ideological conformity is gained when cadres explain to peasants how all among them suffer from continued population growth. For example, when a commune member in the Fifth Production Team of Hexing Production Brigade had only a single daughter, she was well cared for. People called her 'Little Darling'. When this child was five years old, a second child was born. Household chores increased, and there was no time to look after the children. The older child got lice, but no one did anything about it. Little Darling turned into a 'Louse Nest'. This tale portrays how the only child benefits from increased attention in a rural household that is always faced with many productive and household tasks, and emphasize discrimination and lack of distributive justice within a household as a result of its bearing too many off-spring [134].

Other fears expressed are whether or not those who have numerous children are likely to become prosperous ahead of the others. The Dayi county collectives analyze the current incomes of families of different sizes and conclude that households with a high dependency ratio earn less than those with few children. Peasants then ask "whether house-holds with numerous children will become prosperous ahead of others once the babies have grown up?" The reply is

not necessarily . . . because once children reach 17 or 18, though they can make work-points and increase earnings, this is the time when one has to be concerned about getting a wife for one's sons, about building a house, about buying household items, and sending betrothal gifts, all of which require the spending of a lot of money. For male child to marry, the whole family has to save up bit by bit for many years to make ready. If one has two or three males, the expenditure is even greater [134].

A stringent system of birth limitation is seen as socially just if the program benefits the same families whose rights are being denied. In China, the time frame is at issue. Indeed, Chinese critics of the measures have been quoted in the Hong Kong press as objecting to the single-child family policy on these grounds. They complain about the excessive speed and compulsion entailed to limit families to one child in a quest for instant results. They suggest that the disregard for objective realities and possibilities is an expression of 'leftism'. These critics further maintain that holding this generation responsible for all the debts incurred by the several preceding generations imposes too heavy a burden [72]. In Liaoning province, cadres "even believe that the long-range interests and the immediate interests of birth control are irreconcilable" [67].

Collectives counter such arguments with statements on the theme of responsibility to future generations: "If we fail to have a tight grip on the task of population control now, we shall be cursed and spat at by other descendants in the future". Cadres appeal to peasants' concern for their future progeny explicitly, stating, "Our forefathers said, 'Reserve a small piece of land for one's own descendants to plow'. But if we do not strictly control population growth, where can our descendants plow?" [37, 68].

Still others deny that parents of a single child will suffer at all. In the short run such parents are better off. In the long run, the collective economy will prosper from low population growth rates, and if the collective benefits, then families will also. This can only occur if funds that are now diverted to support needy families with many children and the services to these children are devoted instead to capital inputs. Collectives also plan to channel their savings to capital investment and sideline production. Economic diversification and mechanization in turn will expand the numbers and types of jobs and improve collective income. Richer communes can invest in reserve and welfare funds, further benefitting their families. Thus, the fruits of compliance will be used locally [85].

It is clear that in the short term families who limit their births can be convinced that their children are costly [70]. In the longer time frame, however, the rural family may fear that in its own lifetime it will become impoverished if it bears no more than a pair of children, especially if these are daughters. The stress on the family as the key productive unit, a longstanding reality which gains further support from the new modernization policies, suggests that peasants will wish to use all available labor to make fullest use of the private initiatives. There is a contradiction between the economic fate of each family and the collective at present. By the next stage of its family cycle, these parents may have second thoughts.

Although local units commit themselves to help families that suffer from their policies at a later date, the new productive responsibility system militates against success. The local leaders tell the people that by deploying savings from the reduced birth rates to agricultural mechanization within two decades, the need for many hands in the household may be obviated. If not, social services can support families that complied and help them raise their living standard.

It remains to be seen whether these promises can be fulfilled. Couples that lack a child to work alongside them at present, and those without children to support them when they can no longer toil in the fields, need support. However, even in model areas such social welfare support often does not exist [20, 70]. Moreover, the proportion of collective income diverted to the public welfare fund from which old age homes and other support for the elderly come, has dropped drastically ([114], p. 200). Without assurance that their collectives can compensate for their lack of labor power, peasants may not willingly comply.

When we turn to the status of women under the new birth limitation regulations, the picture is not entirely positive either. In Shifang county, Sichuan, cadres feel the need to utilize women's labor more efficiently, but find women devote their 'best' productive years to bearing and raising children. The cadres and analysts that write the study of Shifang take for granted women's home burdens. They assume women will continue to perform housework and that there is no possible substitute for a mother. Two options then face the collective:

both socialization of housework and encouragement of family planning can help change this irrational state of affairs. A comparison of the two measures shows that family planning is more practical because it takes time to socialize housework and turn it into a public utility enterprise. Moreover, socializing housework is no substitute for women's psychological burden in childbearing and nursing. . . . By deeply promoting family planning and putting the childbearing initiative in the hands of women, women can be released from household chores and take part in social work, production and study.

Then women can truly enjoy the same rights as men [70].

But it is not clear that childbearing initiative is in the hands of women, as claimed. In the past, women's status turned on bearing male offspring, which now conflicts with the new standards of small families. In some areas, women are now blamed by their kin if their single-child allotment does not issue any sons. The new marriage law stresses bilaterality of the family and throws legal support behind women in this way. But there must be a material basis for bilaterality [54, 133, 144].

One looks to the realm of payment and promotion of women in the collective for the law to have any meaning. One model collective deliberately attempted to raise women's labor points to the level of men (although the details were not reported) to reward women for labor force participation [70]. However, now that labor points are no longer issued in this manner, strength and skills continue to be crucial for the family productive economy. Since women still marry out of the village, their parents may still be reluctant to invest in their higher skill levels. Thus, it remains to be seen whether improvements in women's standing are forthcoming [117].

In contrast to this, the press reports a surge in female infanticide. We have no way of linking infanticide unequivocally with the loss of the right to reproduce, since infanticide may have been endemic before the new policies. Further, the sex ratios by single age (from birth to age five) published from a 1982 sample investigation show a normal male/female ratio. Local areas might, however, practice infanticide and their sex ratios might be masked in overall figures. The publication of these accusations in China shows that a substantial body of opinion either objects to enforcing an unpopular policy, or warns how much re-education will be needed. If infanticide indeed results from the confluence of the production responsibility system and one child per family policy, it reflects poorly on the social justice of the measures [52, 97, 137, 144].

Political Issues

The new rural economic and reproductive policies that at once decen-
tralize production and centralize birth decisions sharpen political contradictions that previously were either latent or locally resolved. This is
the conflict between the peasants' current calculation of their need for
strong labor power for the family productive economy, and the collective's calculation of the benefits of lower population growth for all. By
acceding to peasant desires to deploy their labor to gain profits, yet
withdrawing the right to increase labor power for higher profits, the
state heightens a keen dilemma. Gaining and losing rights to reproduce can be seen as an exchange between peasants and the collective.
Both policies must succeed. Yet it is also possible that the success of one
set of policies will be at the expense of the other set. This contradiction
underlies the desperation of peasants wishing sons to maintain the
family economy on the one hand, and the collectives' resort to compulsion to gain compliance to birth control policies on the other. The thrust
of this paper's findings is that if, as is possible, the contradiction cannot
be resolved, a political crisis will ensue: the legitimacy of the birth
limitation policies or the leadership itself will come into question.

Observers of beyond-family planning campaigns see them as politically equitable if they have attempted the 'stepladder' approach. If
other less severe measures have already been attempted, stringent
policies may be more justified. The Chinese press has attempted to
locate a political heritage for these stringent policies. Some cite the
longstanding policies of controlled migration as a precedent of current
population control. Further, the leadership did attempt to limit family
size in less rigorous ways before the present campaign. In 1971 parents
with three or more children were 'urged to limit their births'. Soon
afterwards came campaigns for later marriage, delay in the first birth,
spacing of pregnancies and fewer births. But only in 1979 were collective
incentives levelled behind small families. The leadership argues that
earlier efforts had a measurable effect on the birth rate. The 1982
sample survey of 0.1% of the population documents a drop in the total
fertility rate from 4.0 in the 1970's to 2.6 in 1981. But these new low
rates, comparable to Western nations, are deemed inadequate to the
task of achieving zero population growth. Leaders argue that the campaign need not be permanent. In some 60 to 80 years families can again
bear two children, and less severe sanctions will be in force. However, if

such intensive and coercive efforts must be used to enforce these policies, it does not seem that the political or economic groundwork has been laid by previous 'stepladder' measures [3, 13, 14, 70, 94].

Fertility control programs are also viewed as more equitable if they expand options for parents to limit their families. The 'cafeteria' approach is implied: increased choice and provision of a range of methods to reduce family size. There is a lack of observer agreement on the ability of the Chinese manufacturing community to supply contraceptives widely to the rural populace, although urbanites are better equipped. Reports from a Fujian village indicate that the sole means of birth control there in the late 1970's were abortions and sterilizations. Later, visits to the same village found that the I.U.D. and other devices had become available. Increased access to contraception in rural China is a benefit of the present campaign, although the press comments that materials are still in short supply. Nevertheless, the improved opportunity to use an effective birth control method of one's choice, as implied by the cafeteria approach does not do justice to the current Chinese scene. There is immense pressure for parents of two children to undergo contraceptive sterilization, and there is little option not to use birth control, so that expanded options is an inappropriate concept [38].

It is also argued that incentives are more ethical if nonconformists are not unduly penalized [3]. However, it is clear that the entire structure of the birth control policies turns on uniform compliance in China. Leaders believe that the campaign will fail if the number of nonconformists exceeds conformists. Collective living standards will suffer, and only the noncompliant parents with strong family structures will benefit from the productive responsibility system. The rest who complied will feel tricked. This view further promotes uniform coercion.

Birth control policies are similarly assessed against the standard of universal application [3]. Measures are seen as more just if everyone is compelled to comply. Local residents appear to agree. For example, only a minority responded to campaigns in the early 1970's to ligate or abort a pregnancy. When the campaigns ended, those that conformed regretted their actions. People have spoken in favor of the enactment of laws to demand one-child families, so that everyone is compelled to obey. Immense peer pressure appears to flow from the competition of families for fruits from the collective. Families must believe that either everyone or no one must obey in the interests of equity [83, 91].

Slippage and favoritism is yet another issue that may limit the fairness of such a set of policies [3]. Far from being able to avoid compliance with the single child policy, China's elite must adhere even more closely to the policies. Compliance is a barometer of legitimacy to lead. Indeed, cadres in past campaigns were most likely to respond to the call for small families [83], and today, statements are found in the press that rural cadres, PLA units and other leaders must themselves set examples by reducing their size [35, 36, 41, 42, 91].

In rural China, of all ways in which the fairness of the single-child population policy can be assessed, the overriding concern is the protection of the family. Families are most concerned with perpetuating themselves and being able to survive economically with few children. They also do not wish to lose out while other kin groups in the same collective unit succeed. The right to reproduce entails family, not individual, rights. It is on the basis of the survival of the peasant subsistence level that the political legitimacy of the groups proposing the measures will be judged in the future.

URBAN AREAS

Economy

Urban units also promote the single-child family. While urban production units do not directly suffer from population growth, they are reminded by the press that the overall rate of state investment can be increased if population growth drops. With fewer births, mass livelihood can more quickly improve. For example, it will take a shorter time for workers to receive one grade raise in pay if the state saves funds from a lower population growth rate. This is an effort to link short-term interests of factories with long-term state concerns, and so to convince factory leadership to promote the one child per family campaign [49].

Urban units do suffer from rapid population growth in the realm of social services. State units that supply housing, day care and other services to their workers will have a larger bill to pay if there are more children born. They will pay more for maternity leave and lose the productivity of the woman worker so long as the birth rate is high. Factories are also pressured by the workers to give preference to their dependents for jobs. If each worker has only one child, such pressure can more easily be met.

Thus, couples pledge their intention not to bear more than one child. Some obtain wage hikes. Most urban units have withdrawn housing priority to large families and instead extend priority to small families. Parents have been promised consideration for their only child in school and job assignments. Some factories, service and educational units permit workers to retire early and to pass their jobs to one child, and the only child gains priority. In Shanghai, single children receive a monthly allowance of five yuan from birth until age 16, which is paid equally by both parents' units. Still other units promise single children free medical care and education through high school. Yet other units offer only one or two of these benefits. Less profitable factories, commercial enterprises and units as schools and administrative organizations can only provide health care benefits because they have no budget for family planning, from which these perks are drawn. Some units apply the general welfare fund to pay the health expenses of single children, bonuses for induced abortion, sterilization, and food supplements afterwards. The size of the fund varies by enterprise [91].

If a second child is born, the advantages are rescinded and sanctions applied. Wages may be docked, promotions deferred, paid maternity leave denied and grain rations reduced. Productive units have some power to enforce these sanctions since people obtain rations and services like nursery school care from their work units [14, 86, 91].

These measures may create some hardships for parents that choose not to comply. Those that do comply are not faced with the severe economic choice described for their rural counterparts. Workers that have access to state jobs or jobs in collective units that are prosperous do not depend on the family wage economy in which the income of several grown children is required for survival. Thus, urban families with access to state services through their units need not suffer from compliance to the one-child policy.

Social Justice

Urban parents appear to judge the policies in terms of distributive justice. They bargain for improved returns for acquiescence. They express their concern for a fair exchange compared with other urbanites situated in similar positions. The issue is the distribution of rewards, rather than the right to survive or prosper. Competition and bargaining is thus reported to prevail in urban centers [126].

Some urban units cannot afford to pay high perquisites for the single-child family. Even if they offer such subsidies as free education through senior high school, the units cannot ensure the availability of school places. Finally, there are conflicting interests in the urban units. Workers needing subsidies and single-child parents must often draw from the same welfare fund. This sets workers against each other, and reduces the social force for conformity in the unit.

According to a study in Hofei, the capital of Anhwei province, urban couples that opt for a single-child certificate are disproportionately those who already have a son, and those with higher social standing and schooling. Ordinary working-class parents are less likely to agree to stop at one child. When asked their views of the new policy, noncompliant parents express their concern that the policy will not persist. They do not wish to be the only ones to comply. The universality of the measures, then, is a concern of those affected [91].

Universality for urban parents refers also to the nature of the material benefits for compliance. Urban parents are quite aware of rewards available to others in their city. They make invidious comparisons with other parents who receive more material goods and better services for compliance than they do. This point was crucial in provoking opposition to the single-child certificate. These parents invoked the "norm of fairness" [5, 91].

The control by local units over the benefits for compliance to single-child policies means that the level of benefits depends on the unit's resources. For example, units promise better housing if parents have one child only, but the parents believe this promise will not materialize. Still others fear that the government will later extend the benefits to parents with two children as well. Thus, parents in cities request that the state 'legislate' a single-child 'family planning law'. Such a law will deepen confidence that the promised material incentives will be provided. Urban parents are thus eager to bargain for better and more consistent treatment before they sign the single-child certificate [91].

Competition between urban groups in different life cycle stages and with different needs over scarce welfare funds creates some conflict. Some urbanites who receive welfare support because of poverty complain that the incentives are being paid from their welfare fund. They feel they are being denied their just rights [91]. In urban centers, the lack of a direct link between low population growth and resources of the productive unit appears to intensify the jockeying for the right to benefit from compliance to the new measures.

Political Issues

Urban work units, especially the state sector, hold considerable control over a wide range of needs of the workers: from housing, medical care and social security, to other services and facilities. The broad range of needs for which state enterprise are a primary source of satisfaction has given rise to "a form of property rights" over employees ([125], p. 56). This characteristic feature of the urban way of life for a sizable sector is a way of replacing the wide range of otherwise family-provided livelihood elements through the pay check. State sector employment thus reduces the self sufficiency of employees and reduces the need of employees to look to their household economies to provide many needs. Such a form of political economy appears consistent with the reduction of the household wage economy for the urbanites. Indeed, the elite of the working class in the state sector have less need to depend on a sizable family than the workers in non-elite positions (collective and neighborhood units). For this elite sector, then, the new single-child policies do not contradict the organization of their livelihood, and no political crisis can be expected to ensue.

Those in non-elite positions, insofar as they do depend on a family wage economy, may suffer from smaller families. The different family economies of the urbanites thus need further study.

The political criterion of the 'stepladder' approach is relevant in urban areas [3]. Here, beginning in the 1950's, units drew up family size plans for their members when birth control campaigns were in force [102]. There was and is also a wide range of birth control choices for the urbanites than the rural populace [25, 100]. But an individual cannot legitimately decide against early use of birth control.

SUMMARY

We followed the shift in reproductive rights and control over reproduction by the peasant families and their kin of the pre-1949, post-1949 and 1970 time periods, to the post-1979 assertion of political leadership/ collective control over family size. The stage of 'individual' rights was bypassed in rural and urban areas.

In the first three decades of the PRC the rural kin group lost control over productive property, but continued its right to manage labor. This had pronatalist implications. In the fourth decade the collective returned some rights to manage productive property to the kin group, but wrested away the right to reproduce in an attempt to sever the link between material living standards and family size.

Chinese birth control policies are politically inspired and may not rest on a solid material foundation. Although it might be believed that the leadership has the power to force through policies, regardless of their material basis, there must be a viable exchange for the policies to bear fruit. I have thus asked what kind of exchanges are demanded in rural and urban areas. In the rural areas the loss of the right to reproduce at levels peasants decide upon in exchange for certain rights to produce has led peasants to stress the objective reality of the exchange. They wish to be assured that the kinship group can survive in the new environment of decentralized production and responsibility if they should abide by the new family policy. Until rural families can be convinced that the collective can deliver social services and modernization is around the corner, they will only reluctantly limit their family size. Yet the power of the state to deliver appears to have been undermined. Based on evidence so far, we can only conclude that the leadership is aware of the issues that demand material exchange. But the material basis for a collective alternative to numerous children is not yet in existence. Whether or not the reduction of population growth can precede capital accumulation and aid it to reward peasants for compliance remains a question to be answered.

In the urban areas, the loosening of the family wage economy, and closer dependency of families on their work units seems to provide the material basis for political compliance. A sector of the urban workers does not enjoy the solid perquisites of the state employees, and this sector may have some difficulties doing without a strong family economy.

If the savings from a small family can be directed to promoting the livelihood of the same families that did without in their later stage of the family cycle, then the social justice and political implications of the current measures may be acceptable. But in the current economic decentralized environment, it is not clear that equitable distribution can be assured, which may threaten the legitimacy of the policies and their proponents.

University of Toronto
Ontario, Canada

ACKNOWLEDGEMENTS

I wish to thank Debby Davis-Friedmann, Evelyn Rawski and Andrew Walder for written and oral comments on this work. P. O. Li provided valuable data collection assistance, which is gratefully acknowledged.

BIBLIOGRAPHY

1. Andors, P.: 1983, *The Unfinished Liberation of Chinese Women, 1949–1980*, Indiana University Press, Bloomington, Ind.
2. Barclay, G. W. *et al.*: 1976, 'A Reasessment of the Demography of Traditional Rural China', *Population Index* **42**, 606–35.
3. Berelson, B. and Lieberson, J.: 1979, 'Government Efforts to Influence Fertility: The Ethical Issues', *Population and Development Review* **5**, 581–613.
4. Bianco, L.: 1981, 'Birth Control in China: Local Date and Their Reliability', *The China Quarterly* **85**, 119–37.
5. Blau, P.: 1964, *Exchange and Power in Social Life*, John Wiley & Sons, New York, N.Y.
6. Blecker, M.: 1976, 'Income Distribution in Small Rural Chinese Communities', *The China Quarterly* **68**, 797–816.
7. Buck, David D.: 1978, *Urban Change in China: Politics and Development in Tsinan, Shantung, 1890–1949*, University of Wisconsin Press, Madison, Wis.
8. Buck, J. L.: 1968, *Land Utilization in China*, Paragon Book Reprint, New York, N.Y.
9. Burns, J. P.: 1983, 'The Implementation of Sub-Village Elections in South China, 1979–1982', Paper prepared for the Workshop on Policy Implementation in the Post-Mao Era, Ohio State University, Columbus, Ohio, June 20–24.
10. Chen, C. H. C. and Tyler, C. W.: 1982, 'Demographic Implications of Family Size Alternatives in the People's Republic of China', *The China Quarterly* 89, 65–73.
11. Chen, C. and Hagovsky, O.: 1983, 'Agricultural Responsibility System: An Irresponsible Retreat or A Responsible Readjustment?', paper prepared for the Workshop on Policy Implementation in the Post-Mao Era, Ohio State University, Columbus, Ohio, June 20–24.
12. Chen, N., 1975, 'Economic Modernization in Post-Mao China: Policies, Problems and Prospects', *Chinese Economy Post-Mao*, Vol. 1, U.S. Congress, Joint Economic Committee, 95th Cong., 2nd sess., November.
13. Chen, P. C. and Kols, A.: 1982, 'Population and Birth Planning in the People's Republic of China', *Population Reports*, No. 25, X, J-577-J-618.
14. Chen, P. C.: 1981, 'China's Birth Planning Program', in R. J. Lapham and R. A. Bulatao (eds.), *Research on the Population of China: Proceedings of a Workshop*, National Academy Press, Washington, D.C., pp. 78–90.
15. Cohen, M. L.: 1976, *House United, House Divided: The Chinese Family in Taiwan*, Columbia University Press, New York, N.Y.
16. Cohen, M. L.: 1970, 'Developmental Process in the Chinese Domestic Group', in M. Freedman (ed.), *Family and Kinship in Chinese Society*, Stanford University Press, Stanford, Calif., pp. 21–36.

17. Croll, E.: 1981, *The Politics of Marriage in Contemporary China*, Cambridge University Press, Cambridge, U.K.
18. Croll, E.: n.d., *The Chinese Household and its Economy: Urban and Rural Survey Data*, Queen Elizabeth House, Contemporary China Centre Resource Paper, Oxford, U.K.
19. Croll, E.: 1983, 'Production Versus Reproduction: A Threat to China's Development Strategy', *World Development* **11**, No. 6, 467–81.
20. Davis-Friedmann, D.: 1978, 'Welfare Practice in Rural China', *World Development* **6**, 609–19.
21. Davis-Friedmann, D.: 1981, 'The Chinese Family and the Four Modernizations', in R. B. Oxnam and R. C. Bush (eds.), *China Briefing, 1981*, Westview Press and China Council of Asia Society, New York, N.Y., pp. 76–78.
22. Davis-Friedmann, D.: 'Retirement Practices in China: Recent Developments', mimeo, presented at conference on Aging and Retirement in Cross-Cultural Perspectives, Bellagio, Italy.
23. Diamond, N.: 1975, 'Collectivization, Kinship, and the Status of Women in Rural China', *Bulletin of Concerned Asian Scholars* **7**, 25–32.
24. Diamond, N.: 1983, 'Model Villages and Village Realities', *Modern China* **9**, 163–181.
25. Djerassi, C.: 1974, 'Some Observations on Current Fertility Control in China', *The China Quarterly* **57**, 40–63.
26. Editor: 1982, 'Three Major Rural Problems Currently Meriting Attention', *Zhongguo Nongmin Bao*, February 11, 1.
27. Emerson, J. P.: 1983, 'Urban School-leavers and Unemployment in China', *The China Quarterly* **93**, 1–16.
28. Fei, H.: 1939, *Peasant Life in China: A Field Study of Country Life in the Yangtze Valley*, Routledge & Kegan Paul, London, U.K.
29. Fishkin, J. S.: 1982, 'Justice Between Generations: The Dilemma of Future Interests', *Bowling Green Studies in Applied Philosophy*, 24–33.
30. Freedman, M.: 1958, *Lineage Organization in Southeastern China*, Athlone, London, U.K.
31. Freedman, M.: 1970, 'Introduction', in M. Freedman (ed.), *Family and Kinship in Chinese Society*, Stanford University Press, Stanford, Calif., pp. 1–20.
32. Friedman, E.: 1974, *Backward Toward Revolution: The Chinese Revolutionary Party*, University of California, Berkeley, Calif.
33. Gamble, S. D.: 1968, *Ting Hsien: A North China Rural Community*, Stanford University Press, Stanford, Calif.
34. Gordon, L.: 1977, *Woman's Body, Woman's Right: A Social History of Birth Control in America*, Penguin, Harmondsworth, U.K.
35. Guangzhou Guangdong Provincial Service: 1979, October 29.
36. Guangzhou Guangdong Provincial Service: 1979, December 11.
37. Guangzhou Guangdong Provincial Service: 1983, May 3.
38. Guangzhou Guangdong Provincial Service: 1983, May 14.
39. Gui, S. X.: 1980, 'Population Control and Economic Policies', *Shanghai Shifan Dazue Zuebao* **2**, 16–21.
40. Han, M. X. and Wang, S. X.: 1980, 'A Discussion on Planning Population Growth', *Jilin Shida Zuebao (Zhexue Shehui Kexue Ban)* **2**, 17–22, Changchun, P.R.C.
41. Hangzhou Zhejiang Provincial Service: 1979, November 5.

42. Harbin Heilonjiang Provincial Service: 1979, October 15.
43. *Heilongjiang Ribao*; 1981, 'Population's Natural Growth Rate Drops to 8.64 per Thousand in Heilongjiang', April 8, 1.
44. Hershatter, G.: 1983, 'Flying Hammers, Walking Chisels: The Workers of Santiaoshi', *Modern China* **9**, 4, 387–420.
45. Ho, P.: 1959, *Studies on the Population of China, 1368–1953*, Harvard University Press, Cambridge, Mass.
46. Honig, Emily: 1983, 'The Contract Labor System and Women Workers: Pre-Liberation Cotton Mills of Shanghai', *Modern China* **9**, 421–54.
47. Hu, B. *et al.*: 1981, 'Research and Study on Total Population Target in China', *Xian Jaotong Dazue Xuepao* **2**, 115–25.
48. Hu, C.: 1974, 'The Sexual Revolution in the Kiangsi Soviet', *The China Quarterly* **59**, 477–490.
49. Hu, P. D. et al.: 1980, 'A Discussion of China's Current Population Problem and Ways to Solve it', *Fudan Xuebao* **4**, 11–14, Shanghai, P.R.C.
50. Jacobs, J. B.: 1979, 'A Preliminary Model of Particularistic Ties in Chinese Political Alliances: Kan-ch'ing and Kuan-hsi in a Rural Taiwanese Township', *The China Quarterly* **78**, 237–273.
51. Jacobs, J. B.: 1980, *Local Politics in a Rural Chinese Cultural Setting: A Field Study of Mazu Township, Taiwan*, Contemporary China Centre, Research School of Pacific Studies, Australian National University, Canberra, Australia.
52. Jianguo, L. and Zhang, H. Y.: 1983, 'Infanticide in China', *New York Times*, April 11, op. ed. page.
53. *Jiefang Ribao*: 1981, 'Shanghai Municipality Enforces Certain Rules for Planned Parenthood', August 10, 3.
54. Johnson, K. A.: 1983, *Women, the Family, and Peasant Revolution in China*, University of Chicago Press, Chicago, Ill.
55. Jones, S. M.: 1981, 'Misunderstanding the Chinese Economy – A Review Article', *Journal of Asian Studies* **40**, 539–557.
56. Jones, S. M. and Kuhn, P. A.: 1978, 'Domestic Decline and the Roots of Rebellion', in J. K. Fairbank (ed.), *The Cambridge History of China* **10**, Cambridge University Press, Cambridge, U.K. pp. 107–62.
57. Kane, P.: 1982, 'China: New Focus on Welfare', *People* **9**, 25–6.
58. Klatt, W.: 1983, 'The Staff of Life: Living Standards in China, 1977–81', *The China Quarterly* **93**, 17–51.
59. Kuhn, P. A.: 1975, 'Local Self-Government Under the Republic: Problems of Control, Autonomy and Mobilization', in F. Wakeman, Jr. and C. Grant (eds.), *Conflict and Control in Late Imperial China*, University of California Press, Berkeley, Calif., pp. 257–299.
60. Lamson, H. D.: 1935, 'Differential Reproduction in China', *The Quarterly Review of Biology* **10**, 308–311.
61. Lamson, H. D.: 1931, 'The Effect of Industrialization Upon Village Livelihood', *Chinese Economic Journal* **9**, 1027–77.
62. Lampton, D. M.: 1976, 'Economics, Politics, and the Determinants of Policy Outcomes in China; Post-Cultural Revolution Health Policy', *The Australian and New Zealand Journal of Sociology*, **12**, 43–50.

63. Lardy, N.: 1978, *Economic Growth and Distribution in China,* Cambridge University Press, Cambridge, U.K.
64. Lavely, W. R.: 1982, 'China's Rural Population Statistics at the Local Level', *Population Index,* **38,** 665–77.
65. Lewis, J. L.: 1966, *Leadership in Communist China,* Cornell University Press, Ithaca, N.Y.
66. Li, L. J., 1982, 'Introduction: Food, Famine, and the Chinese State', *Journal of Asian Studies* **XLI,** 687–707.
67. *Liaoning Ribao*: 1981, 'We Must Resolutely Control Population Growth', September 24, 1, Shenyang, P.R.C.
68. Lin, Y. S.: 1980, 'We Must Strictly Control the Increase of Population', *Guangming Ribao,* August 25, 1.
69. Lippitt, V.: 1981, 'The People's Communes and China's New Development Strategy', *Bulletin of Concerned Asian Scholars* **13,** 2–18.
70. Liu, J.: 1980, 'A Preliminary Analysis of a Planned Birth Program in a Chinese Farming Community – A Planned Birth Field Study in Shifang County, Sichuan Province', Population Research Institute, People's University, Beijing, P.R.C.
71. Liu, Z. and Wu, C.P.: 1979, 'Population Growth Control is an Objective Demand of our Country's Social Development', *Red Flag* **8,** 69–74.
72. Lo, M.: 1981, '"Leftism" Has Not Changed, and Pregnancy is a Crime – The Ultra-Leftist Practice of 10 Counties and Municipalities in East Guangdong in Planned Parenthood Work', *Cheng Ming Jih Pao,* July 27, Hong Kong, 1.
73. Mamdani, M.: 1972, *The Myth of Population Control,* Monthly Review Press, New York, N.Y.
74. McCreery, J. L.: 1976, 'Women's Property Rights and Dowry in China and South Asia', *Ethnology* **15,** 163–74.
75. McElderry, A. L.: 1984, 'Historical Background for Chinese Women', Ch. 2 in M. Sheridan and J. W. Salaff (eds.), *Lives: Chinese Working Women,* Indiana University Press, Bloomington, Ind.
76. McGough, J. P.: 1976, 'Marriage and Adoption in Chinese Society with Special Reference to Customary Law', Michigan State University, Department of Anthropology, Ph.D. thesis, East Lansing, Mich.
77. McNicoll, G. and Nag, M.: 1982, 'Population Growth: Current Issues and Strategies', *Center for Policy Studies, Working Papers,* The Population Council, New York, N.Y., No. 79.
78. Meillassoux, C.: 1973, 'The Social Organization of the Peasantry', *Journal of Peasant Studies* **1,** 81–93.
79. Meijer, M. J.: *Marriage Law and Policy in the Chinese People's Republic,* Hong Kong University Press, Hong Kong.
80. Myers, Ramon, H.: 1980, *The Chinese Economy: Past and Present,* Wadsworth, Belmont, Calif.
81. Myers, R. J.: 1970, *The Chinese Peasant Economy,* Harvard University Press, Cambridge, Mass.
82. Nee, V.: 1979, 'Towards a Social Anthropology of the Chinese Revolution', *Bulletin of Concerned Asian Scholars* **11,** 40–50.
83. Nee, V.: 1981, 'Post-Mao Changes in a South China Production Brigade', *Bulletin of Concerned Asian Scholars* **13,** 32–40.

84. *Neimenggu Ribao*: 1981, 'Guyang County Pays Close Attention to Family Planning Work', September 25, 1, Hohhot, Inner Mongolia.
85. Ng, G. B.: 1979, 'The Commune System and Income Inequality in Rural China', *Bulletin of Concerned Asian Scholars* **11**, 51–63.
86. Office of Population Planning: 1982, 'What Punishment Should be Given to Those Who Violate Planned Parenthood? – Questions and Answers Concerning Planned Parenthood, No. 4', *Fujian Ribao*, 3 August, 2.
87. Parish, W. L.: 1981, 'Egalitarianism in Chinese Society', *Problems of Communism* **30**, 37–53.
88. Parish, W. L.: 1981, 'Marriage and Changes in the Family in the People's Republic of China', R. J. Lapham and R. A. Bulatao (eds.), *Research on the Population of China: Proceedings of a Workshop*, National Academy Press, Washington, D.C., pp. 93–120.
89. Parish, W. L. and Whyte, M. K.: 1978, *Village and Family in Contemporary China*, University of Chicago Press, Chicago, Ill.
90. Perry, E. J.: 1983, 'Social Banditry Revisited: The Case of Bailang, A Chinese Brigand', *Modern China* **9**, 355–82.
91. The Population Research Office, Anhui University: 1982, 'A Survey of One-Child Families in Anhui Province, China', *Studies in Family Planning* **13**, 216–21.
92. Potter, J. M.: 1967, 'From Peasants to Rural Proletarians: Social and Economic Change in Rural Communist China', in J. M. Potter, M. N. Diaz, and G. M. Foster (eds.), *Peasant Society: A Reader*, Little Brown & Co. Boston, Mass., pp. 407–19.
93. Potter, S. H.: 1983, 'The Position of Peasants in Modern China's Social Order', *Modern China* **9**, 465–99.
94. Qian Xinzhong: 1983, 'China's Population Policy: Theory and Methods', *Studies in Family Planning* **14**, Part I, 295–301.
95. Raddock, D. M.: 1977, *Political Behavior of Adolescents in China: The Cultural Revolution in Kwangchow*, University of Arizona Press, Tucson, Ariz.
96. Rawski, T. G.: 1982, 'Economic Growth and Integration in Prewar China', University of Toronto-York University, Joint Centre on Modern East Asia, Discussion Paper 5.
97. *Renmin Ribao*: 1983, 'Investigation Conducted by Anhui Provincial Women's Federation Shows the Seriousness of the Situation of Drowning Baby Girls in Rural Areas and the Resulting Disproportion Between Male and Female Babies', April 7, p. 4.
98. Rosen, S.: 1983, 'Restoring Keypoint Secondary Schools in Post-Mao China: The Politics of Competition and Educational Quality, 1978–1983', Paper Prepared for the SSRC Conference on Policy Implementation in Post-Mao China, Ohio State University, Columbus, Ohio, June 20–24.
99. Saith, A.: 1981, 'Economic Incentives for the One-Child Family in Rural China', *The China Quarterly* **87**, 493–500.
100. Salaff, J. W.: 1972, 'Institutionalized Motivation for Fertility Limitation in China', *Population Studies* **26**, 233–62.
101. Salaff, J. W.: 1973, 'The Emerging Conjugal Relationship in the People's Republic of China', *Journal of Marriage and the Family* **35**, 704–17.
102. Salaff, J. W.: 1972, 'Youth, Family, and Political Control in Communist China', Ph.D. thesis, University of California, Berkeley, Calif.

103. Schran, P.: 1961, 'The Structure of Income in Chinese Agriculture', University of California, Department of Economics, Ph.D. thesis, Berkeley, Calif.
104. Scott, J. C.: 1976, *The Moral Economy of the Peasant*, Yale University Press, New Haven, Conn.
105. Shaffer, L. N.: 1983, 'The Chinese Working Class: Comments on Two Articles', *Modern China* **9**, 455–64.
106. Shenyang Liaoning Provincial Service: 1979, July 20.
107. Sheridan, M.: 1984, 'Woman of the Sties', Ch. 13 in M. Sheridan and J. W. Salaff (eds.), *Lives: Chinese Working Women*, Indiana University Press, Bloomington, Ind.
108. Shibutani, T.: 1962, 'Reference Groups and Social Control', in A. Rose (ed.), *Human Behavior and Social Processes: An Interactionist Approach*, Houghton Mifflin, Boston, Mass., pp. 128–47.
109. Shiga, S.: 1978, 'Family Property and the Law of Inheritance in Traditional China', in D. C. Buxbaum (ed.), *Chinese Family Law and Social Change in Historical and Comparative Perspective*, University of Washington Press, Seattle, Wash., pp. 109–50.
110. Shirk, S. L.: 1981, 'Recent Chinese Labour Policies and the Transformation of Industrial Organization in China', *The China Quarterly* **88**, 575–93.
111. Skinner, G. W.: 1964, 'Marketing and Social Structure in Rural China', *Journal of Asian Studies* **24**, Part 1, 3–43.
112. Song, D. Y. *et al.*: 1981, 'Population Forecasting Model and National Population Forecasting', *Ziran Zazhi* **4**, 249–52, Shanghai, PRC.
113. Stacey, J.: 1983, *Patriarchy and Socialist Revolution in China*, University of California Press, Berkeley, Calif.
114. State Statistical Bureau, People's Republic of China: 1982, *Statistical Yearbook of China 1981*, Economic Information & Agency, Hong Kong.
115. Taeuber, I.: 1970, 'The Families of Chinese Farmers', in M. Freedman (ed.), *Family and Kinship in Chinese Society*, Stanford University Press, Stanford Calif., pp. 73–85.
116. Thaxton, R.: 1975, 'Tenants in Revolution: The Tenacity of Traditional Morality', *Modern China* **1**, 323–58.
117. Thaxton, R.: 1983, *China Turned Rightside Up*, Yale University Press, New Haven, Conn.
118. Thaxton, R.: 1981, 'The Peasants of Yaocun: Memories of Exploitation, Injustice and Liberation in a Chinese Village', *The Journal of Peasant Studies* **9**, 3–46.
119. Tien, J. K.: 1968, 'Female Labor in a Cotton Mill', in K. H. Shih (ed.), *China Enters the Machine Age: A Study of Labor in Chinese War Industry*, Greenwood Press, New York, N.Y., pp. 178–95.
120. Tilly, L. and Scott, J.: 1978, *Women Work and Family*, Holt, Rinehart & Winston, New York, N.Y.
121. Tsui, W. Y.: n.d., 'Equity and Disparity in Access to Health Care', Chinese University of Hong Kong, Social Research Centre, Hong Kong.
122. Unger, J.: 1982, *Education Under Mao: Class and Competition in Canton Schools, 1960–1980*, Columbia University Press, New York, N.Y.
123. Vermeer, E. B.: 1982, 'Income Differentials in Rural China', *The China Quarterly*, **89**, 1–33.

134   JANET W. SALAFF

124. Wakeman, F., Jr.: 1975, 'Introduction: The Evolution of Local Control in Late Imperial China', in F. Wakeman, Jr. and C. Grant (eds.), *Conflict and Control in Late Imperial China*, University of California Press, Berkeley, Calif., pp. 1–25.
125. Walder, A. G.: 1983, 'Organized Dependency and Cultures of Authority in Chinese Industry', *Journal of Asian Studies* **43**, 51–76.
126. Walder, A. G.: 1983, 'Wage Reform and the Web of Factory Interests', Paper presented at the Workshop on Policy Implementation in the Post-Mao Era, Ohio State University, Columbus, Ohio, June 20–24.
127. Wang, C. Y. and Chen., Z. G.: 1982, 'Correctly Handle the Question of Marriage and the Family', *Red Flag*, **5**, 37–9.
128. Wang, Y. C.: 1960, 'Western Impact and Social Mobility in China', *American Sociological Review*, **25**, 843–55.
129. White, T.: 1983, 'Implementing the "One-Child-Per Couple" Population Program in Rural China: National Goals and Local Politics', Paper presented at the Workshop on Policy Implementation in the Post-Mao Era, Ohio State University, Columbus, Ohio, June 20–24.
130. Wolf, A. P., and Huang, C. S.: 1980, *Marriage and Adoption in China, 1845–1945*, Stanford University Press, Stanford, Calif.
131. Wolf, E. R.: 1966, *Peasants*, Prentice-Hall, Englewood Cliffs, N.J.
132. Wolf, M.: 1972, *Women and the Family in Rural Taiwan*, Stanford University Press, Stanford, Calif.
133. Wolf, M.: 1982, personal communication, Stanford, Calif.
134. Wu, W. H. *et al.*: 1981, 'How Do Peasants View the Idea of a Married Couple Having Only One Child? – A Survey Done in Dayi County, Sichuan Province,' *Renkou Yanjiu* 4, 45–6, Peking, PRC.
135. Wynn, M.: 1970, *Family Policy*, Penguin, Harmondsworth, U.K.
136. Xinhua: 1983, April 8, Beijing, PRC.
137. Xinhua: 1983, September 23, Beijing, PRC.
138. Xinhua: 1983, August 5, Beijing, PRC.
139. Xinhua: 1983, January 19, Beijing, PRC.
140. Xinhua: 1983, April 15, Beijing, PRC.
141. Xiao, S. H.: 1982, 'How Planned Parenthood Work Should be Carried Out After Implementation of Production Responsibility System in the Rural Areas', *Renkou Yanjiu*, PRC., **3**, 30–2.
142. Yang, M.: 1945, *A Chinese Village*, Columbia University Press, New York, N.Y.
143. Yang, X.: 1983, 'Controlling Population Growth' 'Planned Parenthood, Shandong Style', *Beijing Review* 7, February, 14, 24–6.
144. Zhang, M.: 1982, 'On the Protection of Baby Girls', *Guangming Ribao*, December 30, 2.
145. Zhou, Z. H.: 1980, 'Population Control and the Four Modernizations', *Sichuan Ribao*, July 10, 3.

HANS-MARTIN SASS

RESPONSIBILITIES IN HUMAN REPRODUCTION AND POPULATION POLICY

Only recently has modern technology given us the opportunity to (a) influence population quantity by nonviolent means (population policy), (b) screen and increasingly influence the genetic heritage of the new-born (genetics), and (c) differentiate between recreational and reproductive aspects of human sexuality (contraceptives). These new possibilities call for new forms of responsibility of the *individual* to his or her self-respect, to other fellow humans, to society and to future generations; of *society* to liberties and securities of its members, and to its own rich and cultivated existence and survival; and of *one generation* to the following. It is my thesis that – as in any new area of human activity created by progress in technology – the concept of *Responsibility* rather than of *Rights* is best suited to handle moral and political issues in regard to the application of new technology.

The thesis may be formulated this way: *There are moral responsibilities and contractual obligations to regulate reproduction; the development of a contraceptive ethos would be a most valuable instrument for exercising these new responsibilities.* It will be elaborated in four steps by showing that: (a) any progress in technology increases the need for making ethical choices (i.e., accepting responsibility and eventually enriching life); (b) new responsibilities have to be accepted affirmatively and innovatively; (c) educated individuals and prudent public authorities are responsible for approximating adequacy in quantity and quality of population; (d) extended responsibilities call for new and innovative ethics of sexuality, parenting, population and socializing.

TALKING ABOUT RESPONSIBILITIES

There is a lot of talk about 'rights' in academic and professional debates as well as in public policy and rhetorics – talk about fundamental, natural and contractual rights, alienable and inalienable rights, vested rights, human rights, the right to die, the right to life, animals' and trees' rights, and the right to or not to procreate. The 'right' issues in regard to new reproductive and contraceptive technologies include the rights to or

135

Stuart F. Spicker, William B. Bondeson, and H. Tristram Engelhardt, Jr.
The Contraceptive Ethos, 135–161.

not to procreate or fornicate, and the rights to control or to deny control of procreation or fornication. These 'rights' are interrelated with the 'rights' to or not to have sex, to have sex in various ways, and to care or not to care for one's kin, lover or community. Bearers of rights are, or are claimed to be, families, neighborhoods, clubs or churches, states nations, deceased or future persons, fetuses or the ingredients they are made out of (sperm and unfertilized eggs), and persons, including physicians, psychiatrists and judges, who might or might not have the right to bestow or withdraw the rights to conceive, contracept, bear, guest bear, abort, deliver or be a person.

It is quite easy to get lost in the jungle of rights – of establishing, vesting, claiming, grabbing, stealing and hermeneutizing rights.[1] The Thrasymachos argument ([58], 3366–3369) that those who do not have the power to take or to do whatever they have the power to do, talks about rights in order to undermine those rights which are taken rather than granted. It complicates the situation even more. It blends easily with the Marxist-Leninist and other totalitarian groups' practice of understanding rights as a means to protect privileges of self-bestowed oligarchic groups, as well as with the political rhetoric on rights, especially human rights, which serves the interests of bureaucracies, totalitarian groups, or power states rather than individuals. There is a usefulness in philosophical investigations into the fundamentals and instrumentals of various forms of rights, of talking, claiming or granting rights, and of the unavoidability of an intellectual and political fight in the area of ideological orientation about rights. But for argumentative reasons, moral and political issues of human reproduction will be best dealt with from the aspect of responsibility rather than from the aspect of right.

Consideration of *Responsibility* first will lead to a concept of *Right*, which is related to the set of values *I* personally am willing and able to embody in my life and environment. In setting certain values higher than others, I *respond* to the variety of choices I have in arranging and exercising value preferences. I grant rights to others because not doing so would violate my self-respect by not embodying values in my cultivated environment of which I am part. The widest range of such an environment would be the totality of agents who are or might be in the same situation as I am: persons who are moral agents (i.e., who cannot avoid making choices between what they, their group or we together see as the right or wrong choice regarding the comfortable setting of the chosen or taught set of values, aspirations, goals and preferences). It is here where the ideas of *solidarity* arise, the greatest of which is the idea of the unity of humankind notwithstanding differences in race, age, education, history or geographical location. From this very notion of solidarity we derive the *idées grandes* of universal human rights, constitutional law, government regulation, or self-regulation by individuals and professional, religious, cultural and political groups.

A simple law – and my second thesis – is that *progress in technology and science, increasing our technical capabilities, also increases (fortunately) our responsibilities, our moral capabilities*. It is a great thing that we can – unlike our forefathers – communicate with friends or partners in nearly any part of the world instantly by phone, fight infections with antibiotics, differentiate between sexual and procreative activities, produce, carry and deliver descendants in various ways – whether we be individuals or couples – and overcome general natural limitations or special personal insufficiencies. It is not only the *possibilitas* of possible uses of available or future technology, but the *actualitas* of actually available technology and its actual applications which increases our *responsibilitas*.

The dimensions of responsibility increase in quantity and quality wherever the quantity and quality of choices I can make also increase. The number and quality of choices I have in choosing between A or B, or between a variety of choices, are not only a result of actually available technology, but are also a result of a liberalization and emancipation process which might be related to the increasing availability of technological and civilizational goods, and which has accelerated in Western culture during the last decades. This process of the *emancipation* of the individual out of natural and cultural bondage is also caused by an increased emphasis on the subjective person's responsibility, and causes a further increase in accepting and exercising personal responsibility; the system of modern open societies is built on these dialectical grounds of flexibility in value preferences as interrelated with personal responsibility. In other words: *Technological progress and value pluralism in technological and open societies are pre-conditional for making moral choices* (i.e., for bearing responsibility whether or not we choose to exercise these responsibilities). Even more, favorable conditions in Western industrialized societies not only enable me to choose, but also make it unavoidable for me to choose responsibly (i.e., to choose in response to what I understand to be the goals, values and forms which enrich and cultivate my life and my environment, and make it more enjoyable). As I owe it to myself to make the right choices, I lose my self-respect if I do not. However, as I often do not make the most responsive choices in regard to what I feel and am convinced will be the most adequate way for cultivation and enrichment, I have to do it again and again, adjusting it to myself and my environment.

Responsibility, therefore, is first and foremost a self-communicative process. But as far as the social and natural environment plays an important role in this self-communication, emancipating, education and cultivating process of accepting and exercising responsibility, such a process leads immediately to the recognition that fellow humans are subject to the same responsiveness to goals, choices and forces in their interpersonal and cultural environment. Voltaire, when calling toler-ance the highest law of nature, made the point that, as far as responsi-bility and failure belong to human nature, understanding and exercising the specific human virtue of responsibility is "the endowment of hu-manity" which makes tolerance "the first law of nature" ([69], p. 487). Open and free societies are based on this kind of reciprocity of culti-vated moral and legal responsibilities of their members. Wherever there is a choice because of value pluralism or technological possibility, there is a moral issue, or in the words of Hans Jonas, the person becomes a "member of the moral order, i.e., one who can be moral or immoral" ([30], p. 57). Contrary to Hans Jonas, however, who advocates restric-tive use or no use of certain forms of technology or high technology in specific areas of possible application in cases in which such an applica-tion might result in a severe change of actually given sets of technical possibilities and moral probabilities, I would not recommend restriction in applying technics. On the contrary, I would recommend an *accelera-tion* in applying ethics in the development and establishment of the 'software' of moral and cultural argumentation and implementation. Restrictions never worked and never will work; if pluralistic countries refrain from technological progress and its cultural and moral control and stewardship, the totalitarian states will set the rules of the game of how to exploit and apply technology. There is a well-coined obligation of the agencies of the *res publica* – government, legislation, courts, occupational safety and health agencies, and mandatory systems of insurance – which takes care of possible hazards of new technology or which introduces higher standards of safety in response to new technol-ogy, and these agencies must and will continue to do so. However, as the concept of 'risk' is not just an issue of science and engineering, but an issue of cultural and moral acceptability and prudence as well [46], and as we do not want governmental bodies to paternalistically regulate ethics, culture and lifestyle, we would rather prefer a minimalistic approach in public policy regulations combined with a maximalistic approach in personal responsibility, public moral argumentation, and education in risk awareness and management [62]. My thesis that progress in technology and value diversification causes moral and cultural responsibility leads to a call for *affirmatively accepting and innovatively experiencing moral responsibility* in new areas of technology.

TAKING RESPONSIBILITIES SERIOUSLY

The general concept of responsibility in reproductive issues was introduced 100 years ago by Sir Francis Galton [18], who presented the thesis that by carefully planned parenthood the genetic heritage of the next generation could be refined and enriched intentionally and responsibly. Galton's only scientific instruments were quantitative methods of analysis; he did not know about the most recent breakthroughs in reproductive and contraceptive technologies. But contrary to Darwin, who held that the selection process was caused by natural means or sudden and accidental changes in genetic codes, and contrary to contemporary sociobiologists, who hold that the process of selecting quantity and quality of population is caused by social means such as pressures, institutions and incentives [71], Galton and Huxley related the availability of scientific methods to the moral responsibility to use such methods which were fundamental for the future of families, nations and mankind in general [28]. This is the special application of the general rule that technical and scientific possibilities create the platform for personal responsibility and political ethics. Among the technological possibilities now or soon to be available at low risk are *reproductive methods* such as gene splicing, cloning, in-vitro fertilization, artificial insemination, surrogate motherhood, genetic screening and preservation techniques for shelving human reproductive material and for freezing early stages of human life [19, 36, 64], and *contraceptive methods* such as condoms, spermicides, intra-uterine devices, ovulation inhibitors or detectors, and irreversible or reversible male or female sterilization [11, 19]. The availability of any one of these technologies, and even more, the combination of them, provide a challenge for responsible stewardship toward new possibilities of enriching life, culture and moral capabilities in the present and future. This is a challenge to the educated individual, to religious and cultural groups in society, to governments and to the international community.

In regard to the diversity of cultures, different political issues in different countries, and pluralism in value preferences in at least some of the more fortunate countries, the establishment of a common basis for moral and political argumentation on how to analyze, accept and exercise responsibility in human reproduction is one of the most crucial issues for both international dialogue and responsible decision-making processes of governments and individuals. Who shall, and by which means and in what capacity, protect, grant, limit, accept and exercise reproductive and contraceptive responsibilities? Accepting the plurality of this world as a rich and valuable heritage, as opposed to uniformity, requires the use of systems of reference which are sensitive to the diversity of cultures and value preferences. This does not mean that different value systems will necessarily lead to different solutions to responsibly mastering and stewarding technical possibilities and to establishing national and international communities in approximating mutual acceptability or tolerability. The fact that different cultural and religious systems of reference may take the same or similar practical actions and goals in public policy or personal moral concern has already been mentioned by the classical theories of the 18th century enlightenment [35, 40].[2] The compromise approach has become one of the major platforms for achieving agreements or acceptance in domestic and foreign affairs where no material consensus of the values involved could be achieved.

The epistemological and methodological instruments for such an approach in population policy is developed by Berelson and Lieberson ([5], p. 45). They adopt "a contextual and piecemeal approach to the ethical concerns which view ethics as a species of decision-making, resting on agreed-upon premises and proceeding to substantive conclusions as to what sort of action should be taken in particular situations." Given the actual international power politics, any inter-governmental agreement in regard to contraceptive and reproductive policies must rest on such a formal basis. So does the international discussion, which cannot restrict its arguments to any one of the cultural or religious traditions. Berelson's and Lieberson's model analyzes five forms of possible governmental intervention into the reproductive decision-making processes of individuals: (1) manipulating public and private access to means and methods of fertility control; (2) indirectly changing fertility behavior by changing socio-economic determinants of fertility behavior such as education, literacy, mortality and life expectancy, industrialization, urbanization, income structure, taxation, status of women and housing; (3) propagandizing governmental views and limiting opposite views, manipulating incentives or disincentives such as "child assistance stipends, maternity leaves and costs, tax benefits, direct monetary subsidies to individual families for 'correct' fertility behavior" (i.e., fees for vasectomies); (4) "establishing community incentives or disincentives for 'correct' fertility behavior" (i.e., roads or schools); and finally, (5) "direct sanctions, from minimum age at marriage to limits on family size" ([4]; p. 77, [5]; p. 2). As private decisions about reproduction are different and related to various cultural, religious and social factors, the res publica, in the best interest of each and any citizen, has the right to regulate, control or suppress by educational incentive and slight disincentive means first, but thereafter, if these means are not efficient enough, by measures more intrusive into the value systems of the citizens. Berelson and Lieberson speculate about the degree of intrusiveness in certain forms of governmental fertility regulations and other forms of regulation such as progressive income tax, gasoline availability and nuclear energy plants. To this list can be added the so-called social-contract programs like Social Security, Medicare and Medicaid. Lieberson and Berelson argue that there is a right to – or better and more powerfully put – a responsibility of the government for reproductive and population policy: wherever there seems to be a need for such a policy, milder forms of persuasion or incentives are preferable first, but stronger forms of disincentives may be necessary.

As the risk-means analysis and the risk management always involve a multitude of factors, most of them related to value preferences, the political decision-making process is not easy; but it is never easy, neither in issues of national defense, unemployment policy, nor in issues of fertility policy. We agree with Berelson and Lieberson when they state that in open societies citizens can fight back more easily against governmental policy, and contribute their input into public policy on a great variety of levels and at more stages of public policy implementation than in nondemocratic countries ([5], p. 47). We do not agree, however, when they introduce their model as not presupposing an "overriding 'correct' ethical system or universally 'approved' ranking of human rights" ([5], p. 30). The system they introduce is the system of arguing freely about conflicts between preferences among ethical values and between ethical values and values of other kinds, and making political decisions based on a mix of rights, laws, votes, cultural fashions and procedural preferences. This is the moral and legal framework of the *open society*, granting individuals and groups *liberty* to choose, enjoy and embody what they want, while at the same time limiting such liberty on a contractual or administrative basis in order to grant each citizen the cultivated and protected enjoyment of his or her liberty, thus providing *security* together with liberty. John Locke's concept of a state of enforceable formal law, enframing a pluralistic society and providing the optimal and interconnected realization of liberty and security in domestic and foreign affairs is, indeed, the best available conceptual foundation which attracts: (a) the majority of educated citizens within an open society, because of its low cost high benefit decision-making, (b) politicians with different domestic and international population policy backgrounds, thus transforming Locke's 17th century British model into 20th century global politics.[3]

While there is still a long way to go nationally and globally to install the *responsible individual* as the central moral and political agent, the very idea of responsible individualism is the only platform to discuss matters such as reproductive and contraceptive ethics and population policy among educated citizens and nations which have or claim to have subscribed to the Declarations of the United Nations on human rights. Such a philosophical and political foundation requires (a) an open-minded, step-by-step decision-making process when dealing with ethical issues, favoring initiatives and actions taken by freely-acting educated citizens; (b) a prudent and fair international dialogue, contributing to responsible behavior in reproduction and education; (c) the right of the government to pursue more severe actions against citizens or certain groups; and (d) the right of the global community to protect itself against excessive fertility activities of certain nations, in case those citizens, groups or nations do not play according to the rules which give all parties involved the most liberty and security.

There was no effective method available in Locke's time to differentiate between recreational sexuality and fertility as he differentiated between religious beliefs with and without practical consequences ([39], p. 78). Now we can; we differentiate between cultivated forms of *recreational and unitive sexual activities without practical consequences* to the quantity or quality of the population, and technology-assisted and non-technology-assisted forms of *procreative activities with practical consequences* to the quantity and quality of the population.[4] If someone or some group within a society decides – for whatever reasons – that he/she/they will not make such a technically possible separation between sexual acts and procreative acts, then their procreative-sexual acts fall under the category of individual acts which *include* practical consequences for the res publica. If the res publica understands such activities to be a threat to it or its citizens' well-being or existence, then the res publica has the responsibility to put such activities under various forms of penalty. This is not a direct attack on the liberty to enjoy unitive and recreational sex, but is an indirect attack on those forms of sex which are inseparably connected to procreation.

In Locke's model and in subsequent public policy, it was always understood as an indication for the existence of a strong state to *tolerate* activities, which according to the open societies' general basis, does not have a right to exist. Among those groups are those (a) who do not accept "those moral rules which are necessary to the preservation of civil society" ([39], p. 90), (b) who claim "some peculiar prerogative" for their members, while being "in effect opposed to the civil rights of the community" ([39], p. 90), (c) who, while living in one country, "ipso facto, deliver themselves up to the protection and service of another prince" ([39], p. 94), and finally, those (d) who on the basis of their religion or ideology can and will not hold "promises, covenants, and oaths" ([39], p. 94). Locke's model of the open society holds the government responsible for taking action, whenever necessary, against those who undermine the consensus of the peaceable society. It was within this conceptual framework that the First United Nations World Population Conference (Bucharest, 1974) declared:

All couples and individuals have the basic right to decide freely and responsibly the number and spacing of their children and to have the information, education and means to do so; the responsibility of couples and individuals in the exercise of this right takes into account the needs of their living and future children, and their responsibility towards society ([66], p. 11).

This basic right is not biologically or naturally given, but is a socially *granted* right, the responsible exercise of which should be based on *information, education* and *means*; it may not interfere with the responsibilities towards already existing or possible future children and with the responsibilities towards society in general. It also should be mentioned that the Declaration does not only talk about couples but also individuals to which these responsibility-bearing rights are granted.

What would be the benefits to individuals and society if people would responsibly work on influencing the quantity and quality of their children by using the availability of procreative and contraceptive technologies? Among those benefits would be at least (a) a better inter-relationship among the functions of producing, educating and caring for children, (b) fewer cases of unwanted, unloved, aborted or abused children, and fewer children with genetic diseases (e.g., fewer cases which produce nearly unbearable moral burdens to all parties involved), (c) more emancipation of women to responsibly accept pregnancy and motherhood, (d) less injustice and social unrest, an unbalanced increase or decrease in population might result in unjust relations between those having and not having children, and (e) less governmental regulation (which is never a desirable means of control, except when self-regulation, i.e., responsible actions of educated citizens, does not work).

Locke's *Letter on Toleration* served during the last three hundred years as a blueprint for the educated Western world in granting religious, cultural and philosophical pluralism without undermining law, order, culture and a state sufficient to protect the liberty, security and well-being of its citizens against enemies from inside and outside. The United Nations model of procreative and contraceptive responsibilities opens, on the same grounds, the door to new forms of sexual, procreative and social pluralism. It grants the individual the optimum of liberty and responsibility, but reserves the responsibility of the res public "to recommend guidelines for population policies consistent with national values and goals and with internationally recognized principles", and "to encourage the development and good management of appropriate education, training, statistical research, information and health services" ([65], p. 13) in order to safeguard the precondition and further development of such liberty and security for the present and future generation.

While this position calls for individual reproductive responsibility, it is well aware of the underlying public responsibility to safeguard and protect the framework within which such acts of individual responsibility are exercised. There may be other positions, among them those close to Christian, Confucian, Buddhist or Marxian thought, which on their own basis might come close to the present liberal Western position.

Indeed, such mutually shared goals and principles of responsible use of modern reproductive and contraceptive technologies is an indication for the truly humanist and ethical attitude and basis of *any of these positions* in a pluralistic world – in which we all must live together with dignity and responsibility – towards a new reproductive and contraceptive ethos.

REPRODUCTIVE ETHICS AND THE AMBIGUITIES IN GOVERNMENTAL INTERVENTIONS AND DOCTRINAL TEACHINGS

Instead of enumerating the numerous benefits of reproductive and contraceptive technologies for the individual's personal growth, cultural enrichment, health and opportunity to live a life based on responsible and dignified decision-making rather than natural fate, let us look into those areas of conflict which might arise – as they arose in Locke's 17th century model of the open society – between the *individual's free and responsible decision* and the *government's responsibility* to safeguard minimum liberty and security on one side and *ideological or doctrinal teaching* based on fundamentalistic concepts of truth on the other. Truth, especially in religious and metaphysical matters, is a delicate thing and cannot be imposed on anyone by force. It is the principle of the open and peaceable society to grant and protect religious and ideological freedom; religion and ideology in return, however, may not undermine the societal and political base which guarantees its freedoms. As groups, especially those holding fundamentalist concepts of truth, are a greater threat to a prudent governmental stewarding of population development than single individuals, most likely conflicts arise among groups, governments and individuals, or – even worse – between groups in control of government or sharing governmental powers. The first type of conflict arises mostly in pluralistic societies, while the other is typical of totalitarian or semi-totalitarian states.

While the methaphysical and cultural concepts of sex and love are not governmental issues, but rather issues of privacy, personal responsibility and culture, the reproductive outcome of private and personal preferences is both a private and a public matter (e.g., there is a public responsibility to control quantity and quality of population production). As mentioned earlier, such a public and governmental responsibility is not just one of nature or biology (i.e., 'quantity' is, after all, related to specific cultural traditions, technological and economic conditions, and change and stability in life-style, while 'quality' is related to education first, and thereafter to responsibly spacing and genetically and medically treating the next generation). On the other hand, not all issues which are claimed to be public issues requiring governmental intervention and regulation are indeed public issues. In an open society the majority of cases are taken care of by the markets of ideas, fashions, life-styles and economy, with mild governmental incentives utilized once in a while to either encourage or discourage population growth or shrinkage. However, there are extreme cases of rather bizarre reproductive behavior of groups which do not blend in with the open market of attitudes, but instead dominate such a market and therefore cause governmental intervention in the interest of the res publica.

RESPONSIBILITIES AND GOVERNMENTAL INTERVENTION

Under present global conditions the fertility behavior of a group, which might *cause underpopulation*, is tolerable – even favorable from a global point of view. For national reasons, however, such attitudes might threaten the cultural, economic or political survival of a nation, or unbalance existing or desirable population structure. The state, therefore, would feel responsible to safeguard, through a prudent and flexible set of incentives and disincentives, the society and its future by means of encouraging marriages, parenthood, artificial insemination, surrogate motherhood, or new forms of bringing children up in a way which would fit into the specific cultural traditions of that country.[5] The abuse of governmental intervention into the value market which initiates fertility behavior would be biased, granting some nations higher fertility rates than others, and thereby new forms of imperialism, by overstocking global markets with people rather than with guns, cotton or computers.[6] New increasing possibilities for tribalism and racism, that would take advantage of modern reproductive and contraceptive technologies, would be a great threat to the rich diversity of the genetic heritage of the human population. This threat might create new forms of responsibility for protecting, collecting and storing valuable material of human genetic heritage in cases in which entire tribes or populations face genocide. The global community already recognizes such a responsibility in regard to the cultural heritage of mankind.[7] As population consistency, growth or shrinkage do not occur any more just as a result of favorable natural and biological conditions, but as a direct result of culture, science, economy and technology, *the population issue has outgrown natural conditions and spread into responsibility conditions.*

Technically we are able, or soon will be able, to make it a fashionable trend to stop human fertility totally without stopping sexual activity, or to increase population figures of today many-fold within a generation without changing or influencing sexual culture and preferences. Technically it is possible to change world or national economy from consumption to reproduction, as it has been done before from time to time by changing economic goals from welfare promotion to warfare promotion. The technical possibility of zero reproduction or mass reproduction establishes governmental responsibility to regulate reproductive preferences wherever the market forces unbalance a decent relationship between quantity and quality of population, cultural and political values. Interventions in reproductive behavior, however, should be minimal and long range, as this is an area of human life and culture which will accept frequent changes with greater difficulty than frequent tax or traffic regulations. A middle-of-the-road approach to reproductive and contraceptive intervention as a part of population policy has to take into account that we would not be what we are if parents and society had not provided us with genetic, educational, parental and social means and preconditions after we were born. To provide the next generation with at least similar preconditions for life and culture includes our responsibility for (a) providing an educational system which teaches those basic skills and social experiences which are necessary to master the existing social, economic and political order, (b) exposing the young generation to the basic values and roots of our and other cultural traditions so that they may make educated and experienced decisions regarding their value preferences and the embodiment of values in their environment, and (c) providing the next generation with the best possible number and educated fellow humans, which includes the use of responsible procreative and contraceptive techniques.[8]

Such an approach makes it clear that pure statistical data on the quantity of population or population growth does not imply anything, as population policy is aware of the cultural, educational and economic framework as well, in which the quantity of the population is one, but not the most crucial, factor. Among the instruments used by governmental intervention are those which are most productive in affecting the causes which most likely produced unbalanced fertility rates (e.g., *economic incentives* if the reason for having or not having many children are basically rooted in economic preconditions; *social incentives* such as public honors, prestige, placements in career or professional positions if the reasons for having no, few or many children, or sons or daughters, are primarily rooted in social or cultural traditions; and *religious or ideological argumentation* addressing responsibility issues in cases of unfavorable or unacceptable fertility behavior caused by religious or ideological fundamentalism). If, as Salaff reports [60], the reasons for high fertility rates in China were primarily economic, then a flexible approach in offering economic and educational incentives, most importantly forms of health insurance and retirement payments, would be most effective.[9] If, however, the cultural, philosophical or religious considerations encourage an abundance of offspring, or at least one son, the need for more sophisticated educational measures has to be considered, including campaigning to increase responsibility towards the community, setting up goals to compete with those which caused the unbalanced fertility rate, arguing on the grounds of ideology or lifestyle concepts, or from the outside, stressing the more important underlying values, the realization of which would change unacceptable fertility behavior. If in one society the use of contraceptives provides a full sexual life and economic and other life-style benefits for a professional single individual, including health care and retirement benefits, while in another society many children provide the same benefits, then the economy or life-style related actions taken by government to change either one of these attitudes would have to be different. If, however, the decrease in the number of offspring would be a serious threat to traditional forms of socialization and living a cultivated life within large families, then, among the incentives to change such a life-style, there would have to be the introduction of new and truly effective forms of solidarity, socializing and interconnecting, such as the cultivation of solidarity between more distant branches of the smaller family, natives of villages or neighborhoods, co-workers within the workplace or within occupational or recreational organizations.

What one can learn from Salaff's article is that the Chinese government (a) accepts responsibility for influencing fertility behavior for the benefit and well-being of its citizens, (b) makes use of the availability (though at some times and places limited), of contraceptive means, thereby not directly interfering with sexual activities, the suppression of which would be a less acceptable means to reach similar goals, (c) backs up the introduced contraceptive ethos with a mix of economic incentives, which over the years will be improved or refined, as will the contraceptive techniques. It seems that the noninterference of the government (i.e., the governments not taking responsibility for influencing reproductive behavior), is most likely much less morally acceptable. Chinese population policy and contraceptive ethics are a good paradigm for demonstrating how the availability of new technologies first impose new responsibilities on the individual, and thereafter on society and government – responsibilities which have to be accepted and exercised, based on traditional value preferences and social, economic, cultural and political structures.

RESPONSIBILITIES AND RELIGIOUS DOCTRINATION

The open society can be defined by its wide range of tolerance regarding the life-styles and beliefs of its citizens; granting and safeguarding such freedoms is the very purpose of the open and peaceable society. If there is a religious sect which holds that it is a fundamental commandment never to separate the joys of gourmet eating from the intake of food for survival, or to not separate recreative sex from procreative sex for survival of the race, a doctrine holding that gourmet eating is an act of gluttony and forms of sexual activity which do not lead to pregnancy are acts of unnatural perversity, would also have the right to exist and impose certain restrictions on its members. Only if certain attitudes become unfair burdens on society, or threatening to its continuation and balanced development (i.e., in cases where certain eating habits cause health damages, the repair costs of which are shared by those who do not get the enjoyments – if any – out of such extreme behavior, or in cases where certain forms of sexual behavior cause population growth, the cost of which and possible damages to the newborn, the economic, educational, cultural or political systems, may also become a burden to those who do not share the views which lead to such sexual behavior), it is then the responsibility of the *res publica* to do justice equally to all of its citizens. If the society and its citizens, for reasons of *self-respect* and human dignity, do not want to refuse a decent minimum of care to those who, as a result of their fault cannot provide for themselves, (i.e., those who excessively abuse food, drink or drugs, or those who owe their life, but barely anything else, to a sectarian sexual behavior of others), then there should be quite a few instruments developed to avoid unfair burdens on the rest of society. Among those means might be taxation of food or drugs which can cause health damages or mandatory insurance against those damages, or excess taxation on children. On the other hand, groups enjoying activities which might cause harm to others, for reasons of responsibility and in order to avoid governmental intervention, could go the way of self-regulation and take care of the results of their activities using their own people, money and value preference systems. There are certain limits to which a community, for reasons of self-respect and responsibility to its values, traditions and constitutional systems, will bear excessive behavior of some citizens or groups at the cost of *burdening the entire society*.

When addressing the issue of reproductive and sexual ethics, we are not talking about issues of biological or national survival as an end in itself; we are talking about cultivating and dignifying human life in constitutionally organized states and in open, peaceable, rich and diversified societies, whose central acting agent is the responsibly *acting individual*. The acting person, according to Wojtyla, is never "a passive substratus", but is living, becoming and developing in acts of "being-acting-becoming . . . living in each of his acts," permeating "every act with his peculiar character. . . . these forms of dynamism proper to the human person make something of him, and at the same time they – so the speak – make somebody of him" ([72], p. 96f). Such a position emphasizing the responsibility and responsible development of the person suggests to the individual that he or she is highly responsible for his or her sexual and procreative acts, and for the results of reproductive acts, which are not just ordinary products, but become fellow persons to whom they are specially responsible.[10] The person is a moral agent because "morality is the fruit, the homogenetic effect of the causation of the personal ego" ([72], p. 98).

The Roman Catholic church's response to the new possibilities in contraceptive technologies serves as an example of how crucial and unpredictable religious responses can be. In 1963 Pope John set up a commission to study the influence of acceptance of contraceptive technologies on the traditional Christian concept of family and parenthood. A majority of the commission drafted a report expressing a contraceptive ethos and establishing theological and moral arguments sanctioning contraceptive methods in responsible marriage and parenthood [55]. The Commission distinguishes between complete and incomplete human acts. As quite a lot of human acts are not complete in the ideal sense, so 'conjugal acts' are incomplete if they do not result in conception due to

natural reasons or human intervention. The Commission defines contraception as a means to perform conjugal acts "which by intention are
infertile", but are "ordered to the expression of the union of love" ([55],
p. 211). Sexuality is understood not only in terms of procreation, but
also as "a manifestation of self-giving love, directed to the good of the
other person or of the community, while at the same time a new life
cannot be received", (e.g., sex is "a legitimate communication of
persons through gestures proper to the beings composed of the body
and soul with sexual powers" ([55], p. 213). The Commission also calls it
an "obligation of conscience" not to generate offspring, given that we
value "the rights of the already existing child or the right of a future
child"; the "procreative end" of human sexuality is "substantially and
really preserved even when here and now a fertile act is excluded. . . .
Man is the administrator of life and consequently of his own fecundity"
([55], p. 213).

Among the criteria for the ethical use of contraception are interventions which are accomplished "with fewer inconveniences to the subject," which are "more fitting and con-natural", and "more conformed
to the expression of love and respect for the dignity of the partner".
Efficacy is also of high moral value, once the decision to forgo insemination has been made and given the fact that "the rhythm method is very
deficient."[11] Contrary to the report of the majority vote, the *Encyclica
Humanae Vitae* [59], given in the papal authority of "authentic interpre-
ter" of "all the natural law" (i.e., "the law of the gospel" and "the will
of God") ([59], p. 215), stresses "the inseparable connection, willed by
God and unable to be broken by man on his own initiative, between the
two meanings of the conjugal act: the unitive meaning and the procreative meaning" ([59], p. 220f).

The Pope argues that laws of nature, given by God, may not be
changed or manipulated by man: "God has wisely disposed natural laws
and rhythms of fecundity which, of themselves, cause a separation in the
succession of births", therefore, the church, "calling men back to the
observance of the norms of the natural law 'teaches' that every marriage
act must remain open to the transmission of life" ([59], p. 220). While
both the positions of the Papal Commission and the Pope do not have
'scriptural knowledge' handy for quotations, both base their findings on
the *interpretation* of human sexuality and the use of sexuality. While the
Pope holds a biological view, purporting that the sexual act must be
performed without any human interference, the Papal Commission

understands sexual activities to be "human acts" (e.g., acts "for keeping and fostering the essential values of marriage as a community of fruitful love") ([33]; p. 32f, cf. [54]; pp. 226–228), and therefore acts to be governed by nature *and* reason (i.e., through responsible use of sexual capacities for "mutual, corporial and spiritual giving" among spouses as well as for procreative reasons) ([54], p. 228).

It has been mentioned that there is a contradiction between the Papal insistence on magisterial authority in interpreting 'natural law' and 'God's will' on one hand, and the virtue of 'responsible parenthood' on the other hand ([59], p. 219), which is not compatible with pure obedience to doctrinal teaching.[12] The ethical issue of Roman Catholics, therefore, has changed from the *issue of pro- or contra-contraception* to the *issue of obedience versus responsibility*. For the non-Roman Catholic citizens, and for governments in pluralistic societies, the ethical and political issues arise during consideration of how the consequences of Papal teaching can be tolerated and by which means the well-being, culture and existence of the res publica can be protected against this or other religious doctrines which, as a result of their qualitative and quantitative burdens on society, can become a threat to the community. While the Papal teaching only reflects on obedience to 'natural laws', couples and educated citizens, whether Roman Catholic or not, as well as governments and the global community of nations, cannot afford to ignore the question whether or not sexual and procreative activity are separable on moral or ontological grounds (a question of *metaphysical opinion* rather than of *public responsibility*). One has to raise the question of who in the end is to be blamed or fined if behavior based on religious doctrination turns out to be unacceptable to the community: the religious institution or the obedient believer. The complex communication within the Roman Catholic church and its unexpected breakdowns and shifts serve as a paradigm for the ambiguous influence inner-denominational decisions have on society. The development of procreative and contraceptive behavior in Roman Catholic individuals and couples, however, seems to suggest that there is a growing separation between Papal doctrine and practical behavior of Catholics, who find ways of circumventing Papal authority and make decisions according to economic, cultural or religious reasons; they exercise their conscience, thereby blending more comfortably into the open society and decreasing the governmental need for handling excessive behavior of citizens by using harsh measures [48].

THE REPRODUCTIVE ETHOS AND THE CONTRACEPTIVE ETHOS

Understanding the ambiguities in governmental intervention and religious doctrines in regard to the individual's responsibility for making use of the best available technology – here, reproductive and contraceptive technology – it is preferable, according to the concept of the open society and the educated person as the prime moral agent, to leave responsibility for reproduction and contraception to the individual. However, there is definitely a final responsibility for the functioning of the res publica. If its existence and value system is endangered by unbalanced population growth or shrinkage, a population policy has to become active which starts by using the least intrusive means, but may not spare tougher forms of interventions, if required. Religious doctrines and cultural movements may enrich the individual's sense of responsibility and the government's sense of obligation to regulate, in cases where the laissez faire – or nonregulation – would be irresponsible. Unfortunately, these movements may also be counterproductive and complicate the processes of responsible decision making of educated citizens.

As in any area of new technology, procreative and contraceptive technologies require an increase in responsibility, i.e., the development of *a procreative ethos and a contraceptive ethos*, an attitude to responsibly use the availability of new technology. Just as the availability of railroads and telephones resulted in an increased ethos of communicating, so the new procreative and contraceptive technology will lead to new forms of sexual, procreative, population, parenthood and human socialization ethics.

The liberation of lovemaking from fertility consequences provides a unique tool for personal enrichment, interpersonal growth, recreation and enjoyment, but it also opens the door to new forms of sexual exploitation, and less caring in inter-human relations and attitudes. We therefore need a new and innovative approach to *sexual ethics*.

The technical possibility of planning and controlling quality and quantity of offspring creates new responsibilities for parents in regard to the number, genetic heritage, social and educational environment of their children. We, therefore, need a new and innovative approach to *parenthood ethics*.

As human reproduction is no longer exclusively a gift from mother nature, but is also a result of human intervention and technology, according to various preferences, fashions and attitudes, there is a new responsibility of society, government and individuals to provide the following generation(s) with reasonable and manageable conditions which are no less favorable than those which we were given. This is a responsibility we feel we have in return for our own existence and the cultural and economic conditions we were given. Reproductive and contraceptive techniques provide us with the means to do so. We therefore need a new and innovative *population ethics*.

Contraceptive and reproductive techniques also cause new forms of human socialization, making the traditional lifelong, heterosexual child-raising togetherness of a couple merely one among other forms of possible human socialization processes in which lovemaking and child rearing can be enjoyed. New institutions like the homosexual couple with or without an adopted child, the surrogate mother, the single mother and her child, the single father and his child, the individuals or groups raising artificially-created children having no real (e.g., legally binding, genetic) parents, and many other forms of more or less harmonious living conditions in never before experienced forms, already exist, and are already or soon will be tolerated. Such a development might increase the richness of human life in all of its cultivated aspects; it might also destroy it. It is crucial question whether – because of the rapid revolutions in reproductive and contraceptive techniques – we might overstress our moral capacities in coping quickly enough with the new technical possibilities by giving all forms of human socialization equal changes. We might want to slow down the process of developing new forms of human socialization by giving incentives to proven social institutions of lovemaking and child raising (i.e., to *the old-fashioned family*). Recommending such a preferential treatment of already-established traditional institutions for a limited period of time is an act of pragmatic prudence, and should not be confused with Jonas' general quest for staying away from certain forms of technology [31]. The United Nations Conference on World Population was not inconsistent, when in 1974, it stressed on one hand the "basic right of the individual to freely choose," while on the other hand recommended as a policy guideline that, "the family is the basic unit of society and should be protected by appropriate legislation and policy" ([66], p. 11). So it is only stringent when, in analogy to the quest for new ethics of sexuality, parenthood and population, we call for new responsible ways of human socialization, while at the same time protecting the family as the traditional basic unit of rich and strong societies. Nevertheless, we also need a new and innovative *ethic of human socialization*.

Our reflections on the moral aspects of new contraceptive and procreative technologies may be summarized this way: Availability of new technology has to lead to a new ethos of procreation and contraception. Such a new ethos will give rise to new forms of sexual ethics, ethics of parenting, of population and of human socialization. There are no fundamental rights in this world, not even the rights to procreate or contracept, but there are fundamental responsibilities – substantial responsibilities in regard to our self-respect, to human dignity, to our fellow humans, to the res publica and to future generations. In issues of conception or contraception there are no fundamental rights, just substantial responsibilities.

Ruhr-Universität, Bochum,
Federal Republic of Germany
            and
Kennedy Institute of Ethics
Washington, D.C.

ACKNOWLEDGEMENT

This work and others concerning issues in the field of bioethics were made possible by a grant from Volkswagenwerk Stiftung, 1981–1983.

NOTES

[1] An informative summary [45] of the 'Right' discussion introduces a rule-based moral concept of rights, while I will introduce a concept of a closer relationship between right and self-respect.

[2] G. E. Lessing [35] suggests that world religions, while having different dogmatics, could agree on common moral goals and should compete to verify the rightness of their position by struggling for such goals rather than fighting each other, while Voltaire ([69], pp. 482–484) describes how people of various religious, cultural, or political backgrounds can and do cooperate together in the stock exchanges of Amsterdam, Bassa, Surat and London.

[3] The discussion of Locke's model ([40], [61]) of open society has recently been somewhat overdominated by C. B. Macpherson's thesis [41] that the most important and highly debatable cause and result of Locke's tolerance concept was the rise of private property and a politically dominating capitalist class; but Raymund Klibanski ([40], pp. 1–42) and Julius Ebbinghaus ([39], pp. IX–LXIII) stress the overall benefits of Locke's political theory for the processes of liberalization, emancipation, tolerance, mutual understanding and diversity in cultural affairs.

[4] Our thesis, which is based on an epistemological and political theory of educated,

responsible citizens in open societies, clearly confronts the Papal teaching, which is based on the contemporary Papal theological interpretation of the Catholic Christian tradition and which fundamentally holds that there is an "inseparable connection, willed by God and unable to be broken by man on his own initiative, between the two meanings of the conjugal act; the unitive meaning and the procreative meaning" ([59], p. 220f).; cf. also the Roman-Catholic natural law concept in Fuchs, J.: 1984, 'Das Gottesbild und die Moral', in *Stimmen der Zeit*, H6, Herder Freiburg, 363–382.

[5] Incentives used in France, differential population growth rates in countries like France, and change of population in the USSR are described in [1]. See [65] for differential population growth rates in countries like the USSR and for governmental measures taken.

[6] See [7] for the special laws against Jewish citizens in Nazi Germany and incentives in favor of increasing Aryan population fertility.

[7] There are cases of suppressing minority populations and of genocide, of which Biafra [51], or imperialism in Campuchea [63], are only two examples. It would be a global responsibility to use the availability of procreative and storage technology to shelve and preserve the genetic heritage of endangered human populations and to create an Institute of Genetic Human Heritage. Technical facilities would be available and would be improved. Availability of new technology might even create a reproductive responsibility to take precautionary actions in order to protect and safeguard the existence of, and insure no harm to, future generations in response to the possibility of harm to the genetic heritage by pollution genocide, war, and various forms of individual accidents or genetic damage to parents.

[8] There is an extended discussion about whether future individuals have rights ([32, 47, 56]), and whether there is a 'wrongful life' in legal terms ([17], [25]). These questions would be, at least in moral perspective, more comfortably discussed under the concept of 'responsibility' and 'self-respect' of the living generation.

[9] As a last resort, the state Family Planning Commission of the People's Republic of China made sterilization compulsory in certain cases in which couples already had two children. In 1981 almost 30 percent of the birth rate was born to parents having two or more children. The sterilization of one of the parents was not done without the person's consent, however, if consent was not given and contraceptive sterilization could not be done, stiff fines were applied, such as reduction of land grants or monetary penalties [70]. Such a policy of contraceptive sterilization seems to be permissible, as an uncontrolled number of offspring in one family – while other families act responsibly and according to the rules set by the community – is a hardship and an injustice to the community, and places the goals of population policy in jeopardy. Comparing contraceptive sterilization in China with the occupationally-oriented castration of juvenile males for liturgical choral services or for performing the opera seria most likely done without consent of the minors and depriving them of full personal development [26], which occurred in Italy through the early 19th century, shows the enormous difference between the last-resort means of a responsible population policy and the irresponsible, cruel mutilation of children for so-called cultural and religious benefits. The Theological Report of the Papal Commission [54] calls contraceptive sterilization "a drastic and irreversible intervention in a matter of great importance" and wants it to be excluded as a means of avoiding conception. It should be mentioned, however, that the most recent developments in technologies of reversible sterilization ([12], p. 18f) and storing and freezing technologies for sperm and fertilized or unfertilized eggs [53] prior to sterilization, do decrease the possible hardship

of no longer being able to have children after undergoing irreversible contraceptive sterilization.

[10] On the grounds of act phenomenology there is no special responsibility for, or solidarity with, the ingredients or commodities out of which persons are made as a result of procreation (e.g., sperm and eggs). An important question to consider is: When does an individual human start to be a person? During insemination or impregnation, or later after implantation, when the possibility of the egg splitting into twins has passed? After 40 or 90 days, as tradition holds, after delivery, or after sustained and energetic acts of breathing, as other traditions hold? The philosophical position of act phenomenology most likely holds, as does Wojtyla, who is Pope John Paul II, that the act of impregnation or insemination is the act of original becoming, of "initial, original dynamization of the individual being as such", while "all subsequent dynamizations due to any form whatever of the becoming process do play the role of maintaining in existence the already originated being" ([72], p. 96). Finally, however, Wojtyla holds, it is "man's action, his conscious acting which makes him what and who he actually is . . . poses the efficacy or causation proper to man" ([72], p. 98); this only occurs after a couple of years. A morally acceptable proper counterpart to the brain-death definition might be the 50th day post menstruationem as a cut-off date for starting legal and moral responsibilities in the solidary communio animalorum rationalorum.

[11] The Papal Commission mentions that only 60 percent of women have a regular cycle ([55], p. 214). The Commission makes additional points in favor of responsibly using contraception: (1) Regarding abortions which are "more numerous in areas where contraception is neglected", responsible use of contraception goes along the lines of nature, given the fact that thousands upon thousands of sperm become useless and are lost in every act of intercourse, and that of approximately 200 ova present in a woman, perhaps only 15 could be raised to the dignity of human life. Abortion, however, does not regard "the right of an offspring already conceived and living" as 'absolute' as "every human life"; (2) Accepting contraception might prevent oral or anal practices, as those sexual acts do not preserve "the dignity of love nor the dignity of the spouses as humans created in the image of God"; (3) Contraception is only permitted as long as it "favors the stability of the family", therefore, it does not promote extra-marital relations which "lack the sense of complete and irrevocable giving"; (4) Affirming the permissibility of contraception might decrease the rate of masturbation, an act which "negates the intersubjectivity" and "perverts the essential intentionality of sexuality, whereby man is directed out of himself towards another" ([55], p. 162). Fifteen members of the original Commission favored contraception, four opposed; a secret vote on the question: "Is contraception intrinsically wrong?" which included responses by bishops and theologians, resulted in two 'yeses', one 'yes with reservation', nine "nos" and three abstained ([20], p. 162). See [16, 20, and 27] for discussion on the Papal Commission. The original Latin text of the encyclical *Humanae Vitae*, with a translation by Robert Bogan, Commission paper and addresses are in [24], pp. 106–262. A translation of *Humanae Vitae* by NC News Service is in [59].

[12] Some pastoral reflections try to exploit inconsistencies in Papal teaching on natural law and the way the concept of natural law is presented by St. Thomas in slightly different wordings ([16, 33]). They officially criticize the Pope's authoritative teaching, but nevertheless, create some room for responsibly arguing and deciding in favor of contraceptives ([2, 24, 58]) within the realm of the Roman Catholic Church.

BIBLIOGRAPHY

1. Armengaud, A.: 1967, *La Population Francoise au XX Siecle*, Presses Universitaires de France, Paris, France.
2. Baum, S.: 1969, 'The Right to Dissent', in D. Callahn (ed.), *The Catholic Case for Contraception*, Macmillan, New York, N.Y., pp. 71–76.
3. Bayles, M. D.: 1980, *Morality and Population Policy*, University of Alabama Press, University, Ala.
4. Berelson, B.: 1977, 'Path to Fertility Reduction: The Policy Cube', *Family Planning Perspectives* 9, No. 5, 213–219.
5. Berelson, B. and Lieberson, J.: 1979, *Governmental Intervention on Fertility: What is Ethical?*, Center for Policy Studies, Working Paper, No. 48, The Population Council, New York, N.Y.
6. Bergman, S.: 1979, 'Practical Aspects of Banking Patient's Semen for Future Insemination', *Urology* 13, 408–411.
7. Blau, B.: 1965, *Das Ausnahmerecht fuer Juden im Dritten Reich*, 3rd ed., Wochenzeitung für Juden Verlag, Düsseldorf, W. Germany.
8. Brody, B.: 1983, *Ethics and its Applications*, Harcourt Brace Jovanovich, New York, N.Y.
9. Callahan, D. (ed.): 1969, *The Catholic Case for Contraception*, Macmillan, New York, N.Y.
10. Callahan, D.: 1972, 'Ethics and Population Limitation', *Science* 175, 487–494.
11. Camp, S. L. and Green, C. P.: 1978, 'Fertility Control for the Future', *Draper Fund Report*, No. 6, Improving Contraceptive Technology, pp. 14–19.
12. Camp, S. L. and Green, C. P. (eds.): 1978, 'Improving Contraceptive Technology', *Draper Fund Report*, No. 6, Population Crisis Committee, Washington, D.C., pp. 1–30.
13. Camp, S. L. (ed.): 1979, *Population and Development. Hearings of the U.S. House Select Committee on Population*, Draper Fund Report, No. 7, Population Crisis Committee, Washington, D.C.
14. Camp, S. L. (ed.): 1980, *Birth Planning in China*, Draper Fund Report, No. 8.
15. Curran, C. E.: 1969, 'Introduction', in C. E. Curran (ed.), *Contraception: Authority and Dissent*, Herder & Herder, New York, N.Y., pp. 9–15.
16. Curran, C. E.: 1969, 'National Law and Contemporary Moral Theology', in C. E. Curran (ed.), *Contraception: Authority and Dissent*, Herder & Herder, New York.
17. Foutz, J. K.: 1980, 'Wrongful Life: The Right Not to be Born', *Tulane Law Review* 54, 481–499.
18. Galton, J.: 1883, *Inquiry into the Human Faculty and its Development*, Macmillan, London, U.K.
19. Greep, R. O. *et al.* (eds.): 1976, *Reproduction and Human Welfare*, A Review of the Reproductive Sciences and Contraceptive Development, M.I.T. Press, Cambridge, Mass.
20. Grootaers, J.: 1968, 'The Papal Commission. Introductory Note', in P. Harris *et al.* (eds.), *On Human Life*, Burns & Oates, London, U.K., pp. 163–169.
21. Haering, B.: 1969, 'The Encyclical Crisis', in D. Callahan (ed.), *The Catholic Case for Contraception*, Macmillan, New York, N.Y., pp. 77–91.
22. Haering, B.: 1975, 'Some Theological Reflections about the Population Problem', in

Population Problems and Catholic Responsibility, Tilburg University Press, The Netherlands, pp. 156–163.
23. Haering, B.: 1977, *Ethik der Manipulation*, Styria, Graz.
24. Harris, P. *et al.*: 1968, *On Human Life. An Examination of 'Humanae Vitae,'* Burns & Oates, New York, N.Y.
25. Hart, H. L. A. and Honové, A. M.: 1961, 'Causation in the Law', in H. Morris (ed.), *Freedom and Responsibility*, Stanford University Press, Stanford, Calif.
26. Heriot, A.: 1956, *The Castrati in Opera*, Secker-Warburg, London, U.K.
27. Horgen, J.: 1968, 'The History of the Debate', in P. Harris *et al.* (eds.), *On Human Life. An Examination of 'Humanae Vitae'*, Burns & Oates, New York, N.Y., pp. 7–26.
28. Huxley, T. H.: 1901, *Evolution and Ethics and Other Essays*, Macmillan, New York, N.Y.
29. Janssen, L. H. (ed.): 1975, *Population Problems and Catholic Responsibility*, Tilburg University Press, Tilburg, The Netherlands.
30. Jonas, H.: 1976, 'The Concept of Responsibility', in D. Callahan and H. T. Engelhardt (eds.), *The Roots of Ethics*, Plenum, New York, N.Y. and London, U.K., pp. 45–74.
31. Jonas, H.: 1982, *Das Prinzip Verantwortung*, Insel, Frankfurt, W. Germany.
32. Kavka, G. S.: 1982, 'The Paradox of Future Individuals', *Philosophy and Public Affairs* 11, 93–112.
33. Keane, L.: 1968, 'Natural Law and Birth Control', in P. Harris *et al.* (eds.), *On Human Life*, Burns & Oates, London, U.K. pp. 27–44.
34. Lessing, G. E.: 1858, 'Nathan der Weise (1779),' *Gesammelte Werke*, Goeschen, Leipzig 1858, Vol. 3.
35. Lieberson, J.: 1981, 'Review of "Morality and Population Policy, 1980"', by M. D. Bayles, *Population and Development Review* 7, 119–131.
36. Lipkin, M. and Rowley, P. T. (eds.): 1974, *Genetic Responsibility. On Choosing our Children's Genes*, Plenum Press, New York, N.Y.
37. Locke, J.: 1689, *Letter Concerning Toleration*, trans., W. Popple, Avensham Churchill, London, U.K.
38. Locke, J.: 1690, *Two Treaties on Government*, London, U.K.
39. Locke, J.: 1967, *Ein Brief ürber Toleranz*, in J. Ebbinghaus (ed.), Meiner, Hamburg, W. Germany.
40. Locke, J.: 1968, *Epistola de Tolerantia*, in R. Klibanski (ed.), Clarendon Press, Oxford, U.K.
41. McCormick, A.: 1975, 'The Catholic Church and the Population Problem', in L. H. Janssen (ed.), *Population Problems and Catholic Responsibility*, Tilburg University Press, Tilburg, Holland, pp. 139–163.
42. McCormick, A.: 1981, 'Reflections on the Rome Synod on the Family', *International Symposium on Recent Advantages in Fertility*, (unpublished), Buenos Aires, Argentina.
43. McCormick, R.: 1977, *Ambiguity in Moral Choice*, Marquette University Press, Milwaukee, Wis.
44. Macpherson, C. B.: 1964, *The Political Theory of Possessive Individualism*, 2nd ed., Clarendon Press, Oxford, U.K.
45. Martin, R. and Nickel, J. W.: 1980, 'Recent Works on the Concept of Rights', *American Philosophical Quarterly* 17, 165–180.

46. Menkes, J.: 1979, 'Epistemological Issues of Technology Assessment', *Technological Forecasting and Social Change* **15**, 11–23.
47. Morreim, E. H.: 1983, 'Conception and the Concept of Harm', *Journal of Medicine and Philosophy* **8**, 137–159.
48. Murphy, F. X.: 1981, *Catholic Perspectives on Population Issues*, Population Bulletin 35, No. 6, Population Reference Bureau, Washington, D.C.
49. Noonan, J. T., Jr.: 1967, *Contraception. A History of its Treatment by the Catholic Theologians and Canonists*, Mentor-Omega, New York, N.Y.
50. Novak, M.: 1969, 'Frequent, even Daily, Communion', in D. Callahan (ed.), *The Catholic Case for Contraception*, Macmillan, New York, N.Y., pp. 92–102.
51. Nwankwo, A. A. and Ifejika, S. U.: 1970, 'Biafra', *The Making of a Nation*, Praeger, New York, N.Y.
52. Organski, K. F. and Organski, A. F.: 1961, *Population and World Power*, Alfred A. Knopf, New York, N.Y.
53. Packard, V.: 1977, *The People Shapers*, Little, Brown & Company, Boston, Mass.
54. *Papal Commission on the Problems of Marriage and Family: 1966*, 'Theological Report', in P. Harris *et al.* (eds.), *On Human Life*, Burns & Oates, London, U.K., pp. 224–244.
55. *Papal Commission on the Problems of Marriage and Family, Members: 1966*, 'The Argument for Reform', in P. Harris *et al.* (eds.), *On Human Life*, Burns & Oates, London, U.K., pp. 203–215.
56. Parfit, D.: 1982, 'Future Generations: Future Problems', *Philosophy and Public Affairs*, 11, 113–172.
57. Perkins, H. F. *et al.* (eds.): 1934, *A Decade of Progress in Eugenics*, Papers of the Third International Congress in Eugenics, New York, Williams & Wilkins Company, Baltimore, Md.
58. Plato: 1900, 'Respublica', in I. Burnet (ed.), *Platonis Opera*, E. Typographeo Carendonio, Oxford, Vol. 4.
59. Pope Paul VI: 1968, *Encyclica Humanae Vitae*, quoted in the translation of NC News Service, 'Humanae Vitae. On Human Life', in D. Callahan (ed.), *The Catholic Case for Contraception* Macmillan, New York, N.Y., pp. 212–238.
60. Salaff, J.: 1985, 'The Right to Reproduce: The People's Republic of China', in this volume, pp. 89–134.
61. Sass, H. M.: 1978, 'Ideational Politics and the Word Tolerance', *Philosophy and Rhetoric* **11**, 98–113.
62. Sass, H. M.: 1980, 'The Quest for Humanism in a Scientific Society', *Zeitschrift fuer allgemeine Wissenschaftstheorie* **11**, 45–52.
63. Seagrave, St.: 1981, *Yellow Rain. A Journey through the Terror of Chemical Warfare*, Evans and Comp., New York, N.Y.
64. Shinn, R. L.: 1978, 'Gene Therapy: Ethical Issues', in W. Reich (ed.), *Encyclopedia of Bioethics*, The Free Press, New York, N.Y., pp. 521–527.
65. Szporluk, R.: 1971, 'The Nations of the USSR in 1970', *Survey* **17**, no. 4, 67–100.
66. United Nations, Center for Economic and Social Information: 1974, *United Nations World Population Conference. Action Taken at Bucharest*, No. 38575, United Nations, New York, N.Y.
67. United States Congress, Office of Technology Assessment: 1982, *World Population*

and Fertility Planning Technologies: The Next 20 Years, U.S. Government Printing Office, Washington, D.C.
68. Veatch, R. M.: 1977, 'Governmental Population Incentives: Ethical Issues at Stake', *Studies in Family Planning* **8**, No. 4, 100–108.
69. Voltaire, F. M.: 1962, *Philosophical Dictionary*, trans., P. Gray, New York, N.Y.
70. Weisskopf, M.: 1983, 'China Orders Sterilization for Parents', *The Washington Post*, May 28, A1 and A17.
71. Wilson, E. O.: 1975, *Sociobiology. The New Synthesis*, Harvard University Press, Cambridge, Mass.
72. Wojtyla, K.: 1979, *The Acting Person*, D. Reidel Publ. Co., Dordrecht, Holland.

SECTION III

SOCIAL RESPONSIBILITY AND PUBLIC POLICY

NANCY NEVELOFF DUBLER

THE RIGHT TO FORNICATION; THE RIGHT TO REPRODUCE

Mr. Justice Holmes, whose rhetorical and conceptual elegance has scant competition in the annals of American law, observed that: "The law is the witness and external deposit of our moral life. Its history is the history of the moral development of the race" [7]. He also commented that "every important principle which is developed by litigation is in fact and at bottom the result of more or less definitely understood views of public policy; most generally, to be sure . . . the unconscious result of instinctive preferences and inarticulate convictions . . ." [6]. These observations, relevant to all aspects of jurisprudence, are particularly interesting in regard to developments in legislation and case law which address changing patterns of sexual behavior.

The sexual revolution has occurred; it has changed society, been recorded by the press, and exploited by the media. Patterns of sexual conduct have been studied by researchers in the humanities and medicine. There is even talk now about a sexual counter-revolution, a revisionism which recognizes the physical, moral and societal hazards of this newly sanctioned freedom. Increasingly unforeseen biological consequences of sexual license are requiring a new personal calculus of risk and benefit.

Sexuality is profoundly non-rational. It is instinctive and responsive to unconscious desires. Nonetheless, law and public policy regarding this primal drive must be rational and considered. Therein lies one of the interesting tensions of the times. It should therefore be neither surprising nor shocking in this post-Freudian era, juxtaposing Holmesian statements and American sexual practices, that case law holdings and statutes in regard to sexuality are an example of analytic content in some disarray.

Sexuality is a private matter. Patterns of sexual conduct, however, may be of legitimate public concern. For, although there are only individual consequences from discrete sexual acts, societal consequences may attach to patterns of sexual behavior. As our Victorian attitudes towards sexuality have disintegrated, a new schema of statutes controlling sexual conduct and a range of judicial opinions expanding

165

Stuart F. Spicker, William B. Bondeson, and H. Tristram Engelhardt, Jr.
The Contraceptive Ethos, 165 181.
© 1987 *by D. Reidel Publishing Company.*

sexual rights has emerged. But to support sexual freedom while at the same time maintaining some residue of communal morality is a challenge not only for legislatures and judges: all thoughtful persons should contemplate the possible intended and unintended consequences of our new sexual ethos.

Individual passion may be antithetical to regulation. Patterns of sexual behavior however also involve conduct either in concert with or in opposition to majoritarian morality. Some have argued that sexual patterns of behavior either support or threaten the very foundation of society. Since morality has, from ancient times, been considered an appropriate area for legal concern, so may sexual behavior patterns as well.

This paper will address the right to fornicate and the right to reproduce. The first section will explore some aspects of the nature of these rights, and the themes of individual choice and self-determination which they encompass. It will address the development of the doctrine of the right to privacy and the rationales provided for that doctrine in decisions about medical care and sexual behavior. Common elements and themes developed in cases considering issues of contraception, abortion and sterilization will be considered. The second part of this comment will address sexual expression which has not yet fallen squarely within the right to privacy and thus whose adherents exist on the fringe of legal acceptability and criminal prosecution. Finally, a number of problem areas which appear on the horizon will be noted.

The Oxford English Dictionary (under the magnifying glass) produces the following definition of fornication: "Voluntary sexual intercourse between a man (in restricted use, an unmarried man) and an unmarried woman; In Scripture extended to adultery" [12]. The right to follow one's passions and to engage in sexual intercourse outside of the sanctified state of marriage, i.e., to fornicate, has in general been seen as suspect by states following the majoritarian morality of the Judaeo-Christian tradition (although both crown and peasant regularly evaded the prohibition without any subsequent punishment).

In contrast to this traditionally articulated moral and legal norm, the last decades have seen serious challenges to the inherent power of government, secular or theological, to control fornication and the consequences thereof. A set of fundamental and protected constitutional rights, including the right to use contraceptives [18, 21, 24] and the right to control the consequences of one's fornication through the use of abortion [38], has been developed. Women, and by extension men, now have the right to choose "whether to bear or beget a child" [21]. There is thus protection for, and some would argue enshrinement of, the inviolability of individual sexual choice.

Where have these rights come from? How have we moved in the short period of a few decades to a panoply of constitutional protections which have insulated individual action from the imposition of what was theretofore considered quite proper state interest and control?

I would suggest that the answer to this question lies in a parallel examination of those cases establishing the right of persons to consent to or to refuse medical care and treatment. The cases in both areas struggle with the relationship of people to their bodies. In both realms there has been the inexorable march over the last two decades to deify individual decision-making, personal choice, self-determination and autonomy against the opinions, desires and wishes of others. In medicine, the 'others' are skilled caregivers, medical institutions and occasionally family members. In matters of sexuality, the 'others' are the proponents of the articulated majoritarian sexual norms.

This process has not occurred without occasional screams of protest. Exemplary for their rancor and anguish are the remarks of Mr. Justice Rehnquist in his dissent from the opinion extending the right to use contraceptives to minors:

'Those who valiantly but vainly defended the heights of Bunker Hill in 1775 made it possible that men such as James Madison might later sit in the first Congress and draft the Bill of Rights to the Constitution. The post Civil War Congresses which drafted the Civil War Amendments to the Constitution could not have accomplished their task without the blood of brave men on both sides which was shed at Shiloh, Gettysburg, and Cold Harbor. If those responsible for these Amendments, by feats of valor or efforts of draftsmanship, could have lived to know that their efforts had enshrined in the Constitution the right of commercial vendors of contraceptives to peddle them to unmarried minors through such means as window displays and vending machines located in the men's room of truck stops, nothwithstanding the considered judgment of the New York Legislature to the contrary, it is not difficult to imagine their reaction' [18].

Within medicine, concepts of individual control over one's body began with the 1914 statement by Judge Cardozo that, "every human being of adult years and sound mind shall have the right to determine what shall be done with his own body" [41]. That concept of self-determination, which bioethicists over the last decade have explored under the rubric of autonomy, has now been supported by a host of cases which conclude that individual persons applying even idiosyncratic algorithms of strong personal values can weigh and balance personal preferences against suggested medical interventions. The availability of technology and the possible application of medical skill have been recognized as representing offerings for which the acceptance, in the general formula of contract language, must be provided by the individual [17, 19, 26, 34, 40, 46].

Issues of personal preference, ability to withstand pain, financial burden and the emotional environment of the family are all the sorts of values which only an individual patient can inject into, and weigh within, a decision-making process. Thus the doctrine of informed consent, the legal support for individual decision-making, mediates the allocation of responsibility and authority to the individual. This is true despite the very formidable barriers to the application of the doctrine presented by the bias of institutions and caregivers, the state of modern technological medicine and the nature of the consent process itself. It is also true despite the personal disabilities and inabilities, ego-regressed states and timidities of sick persons.

Informed consent provides a fulcrum which permits power to tip to the individual. It permits an individual to accept or to reject an offering of expertise and skill. The doctrine is supported by centuries' old legal theory, which labelled medicine as touching and required consent of the patient as a barrier to a later suit in assault and battery [13]. More recently, the doctrine became grounded in the physician's duty to inform, which is part of his duty to care [17, 19, 26]. Finally, informed consent and its converse right to refuse have been supported by the constitutional 'right to privacy', the very same right which creates protections for choices about sexuality [35, 44].

The 'right to privacy' was enunciated by Justice Brandeis in his seminal dissent in *Olmstead v. United States*, which he stated:

'The makers of our constitution undertook to secure conditions favorable to the pursuit of happiness. They recognized the significance of man's spiritual nature, of his feelings and of his intellect. They knew that only a part of the pain, pleasure and satisfactions in life are to be found in material things. They sought to protect Americans in their belief, their thoughts, their emotions, and their sensations. They conferred, as against the government, the right to be let alone – the most comprehensive of rights and the most valued by civilized men' [29].

This earliest articulation appeared in a case involving civil law. The concept, however, of a sphere of private, personal individual liberty has now come to have constitutional support.

While an appellate justice in the District of Columbia, Justice Burger elaborated on the 'right to be alone'. He stated:

'Nothing in this utterance suggests that Justice Brandeis thought an individual possesses these rights only as to *sensible* beliefs, *valid* thoughts, *reasonable* emotions, or *well-founded* sensations. I suggest he intended to include a great many foolish, unreasonable and even absurd ideas which do not conform, such as refusing medical treatment even at great risk' [33].

The 'right to privacy' is that right which was proposed in *Griswold v. Connecticut* [24] as the supporting constitutional pinion for the protected ability of married persons to use contraceptives. This right of privacy, relied upon in *Griswold v. Connecticut*, and extended to unmarried persons in *Eisentadt v. Baird* [21], established that there is a personal *fundamental* right, granted to individuals and protected by the Fourteenth Amendment, to choose and use contraceptive devices either for sanctified sex or during fornication.

The contours of this right are shaped by growing respect for autonomy and individual choice and by increasing recognition of the private nature of sexuality. One case comments on the intensely personal, almost 'transcendental' quality of the action [30]. All of the cases comment on the impossibility and the unseemliness of the state to enforce criminal prohibitions of private behavior.

In *Einsenstadt v. Baird* [21], the Court held that if married persons were permitted to buy and, by implication, to use contraceptives, the Equal Protection Clause prohibited the state from discriminating against unmarried persons. Mr. Justice Brennan stated for the Court:

'It is true that in *Griswold* the right of privacy in question inhered in the marital relationship. Yet the marital couple is not an independent entity with a mind and heart of its own, but an association of two individuals each with a separate intellectual and emotional makeup. If the right of privacy means anything, it is the right of the *individual*, married or single, to be free from unwarranted governmental intrusion into matters so fundamentally affecting a person as the decision whether to bear or beget a child' [21].

This right of privacy became the basis for the decision of a woman, in conjunction with her physician, to choose an abortion. The first abortion decision [38] and its later refinements [15, 32] established that this right to privacy, which protects individual decisions in regard to forbearance from reproduction, represents the sort of *fundamental* right which the state can restrict only by a clear showing of harm or by demonstration of a compelling state interest [38]. For example, the preservation of potential life after the viability of the fetus has been established is a state interest which surpasses individual choice; at that point the state may prohibit the woman's exercise of her right to abort [38].

The ability of the state to regulate these private and fundamental rights is regarded with constitutional skepticism and held to a standard of strict scrutiny [11]. Any infringement of these rights must be justified by a showing that the regulation is necessary for the accomplishment of an overriding state interest; the harm must be supported by more than mere assertion of its existence. Strict scrutiny ensures that neither majoritarian whim, inarticulate preference nor unfelt assumptions of right or wrong are sufficient to outweigh individual liberties. Thus, personal decisions about reproduction and the moment at which it may occur are protected from state interference or supervision.

Given this legal support, can any logical and rational distinctions be drawn between reproductive and recreational sex? In this arena lies the new skirmish between individual preference and societal paternalism.

Given a fundamental right to use contraception and a woman's fundamental right to choose "whether or not to terminate pregnancy" [38], *is there a right to fornicate?* Moreover, is there an affirmative *right to reproduce* which is as strong as a right to control reproduction? My tentative answer to both would be no. The Supreme Court said specifically in 1977 that:

'Contrary to the suggestion advanced in Mr. Justice Powell's opinion, we do not hold that state regulation must meet this standard 'whenever it implicates sexual freedom,' . . . but only when it 'burden(s) an individual's right to decide to prevent conception or terminate pregnancy by substantially limiting access to the means of effectuating that decision.' As we observe below, 'the Court has not definitively answered the difficult question whether and to what extent the Constitution prohibits state statutes regulating (private consensual sexual) behavior among adults'' [18].

For example, in 1976 the U.S. Supreme Court let stand the case of *Doe v. Commonwealth's Attorney* [20] and thus summarily affirmed the constitutionality of Virginia's Sodomy Law which criminalized various aspects of heterosexual coupling and all homosexual behavior. Evidently individual sexual preference is not all constitutionally protected.

The positive right to reproduce, it may be argued, is even more limited. *Buck v. Bell* [16] (that lapse of Holmesian elegance) produced the phrase 'three generations of imbeciles are enough,' and held that despite some right of persons to reproduce, Carrie Buck posed a threat so serious to her society (in that she might spread her feeblemindedness through her as of yet unborn children), that she could be sterilized by the powers of the state. *Buck* and *Doe v. Commonwealth* thus represent existing law which establishes clear limitations on the right to fornicate and the right to reproduce.

Consider, however, the language in *Skinner v. Oklahoma*, [42], in which the Court, using the appropriate standard of strict review for fundamental rights, struck down an Oklahoma statute which provided for the sterilization of certain habitual criminals. In that case the Court stated that, "marriage and procreation are fundamental to the very existence and survival of the race" and that the ability to have offspring was "a right which is basic to the perpetuation of a race", so that the state could not, in the absence of a definitive and overwhelming showing of harm, destroy these abilities (societal order and police power were not sufficient justification). *Buck v. Bell* and *Skinner v. Oklahoma* are both legacies of the eugenics movement and, in their opposition, reflect the larger debates on the appropriateness of sterilization.

The law now protects the right to choose sterilization and the right to be protected against compulsory or non-consensual sterilization. Thus, physicians may not be prohibited from performing sterilizations [25], and unconsenting persons may not be forced to undergo the procedure [36]. Even more interestingly, capable, competent women, able to give an informed consent, may properly be limited in their exercise of the right to choose sterilization by certain stipulations. Time limits may be set and an educational process imposed to ensure the adequacy of consent [10].

The case which most extensively explored modern sterilization abuses and which documented the ongoing possibility of abuse was *Relf v. Weinberger* [36]. This case involved two young black children ages 12 and 14 who were sterilized without their, or their parents', consent. They were not presented with information as to the nature and consequences of the procedure and the procedure was performed over their objections. (Indeed, one of the sisters escaped sterilization only by locking herself in a closet.) Judge Gaselle, in analyzing statistics on the number of sterilizations, the ages of the children and the race of the children involved, stated that:

'[T]here is uncontroverted evidence in the record that minors and other incompetents have been sterilized with federal funds and that an indefinite number of poor people have been improperly coerced into accepting a sterilization operation under the threat that various federally-supported welfare benefits would be withdrawn unless they submitted to irreversible sterilization' [36].

Despite this case, instances of sterilization abuse have continued to be documented, especially among non-English speaking minority women [4]. For example, consent for sterilization has been requested, in English, by physicians at the time of delivery, despite the fact that Spanish was the mother's language of competence. Such abuse runs counter to the cases which have defined informed consent and mandated that this process precedes medical interventions. It also appears to contradict the assumptions in *Relf v. Weinberger* that sterilizations, especially on poor women, should be free of the fact, or even the aura, of coercion.

The pattern of cases indicates clearly that there is a very strong individual right to *control* reproduction. The affirmative right to reproduce, however, may be undercut either by less than freely considered sterilizations, by improper application of sterilization laws (in my view) or, in some instances, by the permitted application of statutes to the mentally infirm in state institutions. It is encouraging, however, that as the eugenics movement and its assumption of the possibility and desirability of ensuring the purity of the race have fallen into disrepute, the imposition of sterilizations on the unconsenting has markedly declined.

In fact, the climate of the times is such that precisely the opposite problem has emerged as an issue. The case of *Ruby v. Massey* [39] examined the plight of three unrelated girls cared for in part by their parents. The law in Connecticut permitted the sterilization of the incompetent only within state institutions. The parents had applied for institutionalization for all of their daughters. The waiting period was such, however, that places had not yet been provided. The following is the statement of facts from the brief in support of the motion for summary judgment which was presented in this case:

The facts of this case are not in dispute and were set forth in a stipulation filed on July 11, 1977. The stipulation illustrated the compelling personal circumstances of the plaintiffs and gave context to their decision to seek the sterilization of their daughters.

The three girls (Susan age 12, Valerie age 13, and Lynn age 15) are severely mentally retarded and physically handicapped (blind-deaf). Susan and Valerie have no useful communication abilities; Lynn has only minimal ability to communicate. Although at present the girls are residents of a special school during the week, and live with their parents on the weekends, custodial care is inevitable for each of them because of their grossly impaired mental functioning and physical handicaps. The Diamonds have sought Valerie's admission to one of the two state institutions for the retarded since 1968. Priscilla Pearl has sought Lynn's admission since 1970. Neither girl is apt to be admitted to a state institution in the foreseeable future.

Each of the girls shows signs of sexual development. Susan began to menstruate in July, 1975. She suffers severe and painful cramping before and during her menstrual periods, as well as great psychological distress. Susan cannot care for her own hygienic needs during menstruation and it is highly unlikely that she will ever be able to do so. Neither Valerie nor Lynn has begun to menstruate yet but it is equally unlikely that either girl be able to care for her own hygienic needs during menstruation.

The girls are presumably capable of conceiving, but if they were to become pregnant, they would be subject to grave risks because they are incapable of communicating with a physician about their own physical condition – i.e., whether they have had fainting spells, whether they are in pain, whether they can feel the fetus move, whether they are in labor. Moreover, it is most unlikely that any of the girls would ever be able to use, reliably or safely, any of the standard means of contraception. They cannot communicate with a physician about pain they might be suffering from an IUD, from an infection or ectopic pregnancy, and they are unable to check themselves to see if an IUD has been expelled. In terms of preventive health care, the girls cannot be examined internally or tested (for cervical cancer, venereal disease, vaginal infection) without being put under a general anesthetic each time, with all the dangers posed by that process.

In this case the combination of restrictive statutory authority to perform abortions, and a sensitivity to enforced inappropriate sterilizations, had combined to condemn these children to continued sexual potential.

The court in this case eventually permitted the sterilization, as have a number of other state courts. In a New Jersey case [23], for example, the parents of a non-institutionalized, Down's Syndrome, 19 year old female sought the appointment of a guardian authorized to consent to sterilization. Essentially, the New Jersey State Supreme Court stated that the "right to be sterilized", using substituted consent, was included in the range of actions protected by the "right to privacy". It instructed that the trial court be empowered to determine by "clear and convincing evidence" that the sterilization was in the child's *best interest* [23].

The problem with applying doctrines of privacy, which were developed to protect 'choice' to incompetent persons is, I believe, a fatal analytic flaw in these cases. The right to privacy is that right which developed as a support for the right to use contraceptives or to opt for an abortion. The sense in which the right to privacy protects the rights of incompetents to 'choose' is an example of the way in which legal doctrines occasionally expand into adjacent populations and situations, thereby doing violence to coherence, consistency and logic. It may be that the abilities of modern medical technology demand, and common sense dictates, that the law develop a theory to stop the misery of the insensate person. The right to privacy, which preeminently involves choice, was not, in my view, the best legal theory for the purpose. The destruction of the essence of a legal principle is not justified merely by the propriety of the result.

As before noted, the right to fornicate or the right to choose one's sexual partner is also limited by patterns of prosecution in various states, especially in regard to homosexual activity [14]. This is most accurately classified not as fornication but sodomy. The line, however, is unclear, as some heterosexual positioning is also classified as sodomy. It was estimated in the earliest review of American sexual practices by Kinsey that a major portion of all adult males had earlier homosexual experiences [8]. Present estimates indicate that at least 10 to 15% of the American population is attracted to, stimulated by, or sexually gratified by partners of the same sex [9]. For many gay persons, therefore, sexual activity exists without protection of law and is often accompanied by the implicit or explicit harassment by police. The threat of criminal prosecution lurks. Thus, the legal liabilities which may attach to the free exercise of homosexual liaisons and to some heterosexual arrangements are a major barrier to the right to sexual expression for a large part of the population.

Twenty-nine states presently have statutes which prohibit sodomy [14]. Despite puritan references in the legislative history or even in the existing statutes to non-approved heterosexual *positioning*, these statutes are generally assumed to apply to homosexual lovemaking. A recent New York State case [31], however, challenges this general abridgment of homosexual rights and provides a new, logically compelling extension of this application of the right to privacy. The question to be raised about this case is not intellectual consistency, but rather wisdom.

People v. Onofre [31] consolidated issues of heterosexual sodomy with the more politically sensitive issue of homosexual sodomy. The *Onofre* case was a consolidation, on appeal, of three separate cases involving charges of consenting adult homosexual and heterosexual contact.

Onofre was charged by his homosexual lover with forcible sodomy. However, once the accused produced photographs of the alleged acts, the complainant withdrew his charge and admitted that the acts had been part of a consenting relationship. A second case involved two male defendants who were discovered engaged in an act of oral sodomy in a parked automobile at night. The final case involved a woman who was charged with engaging in an act of oral sodomy with a male in a parked truck at night. The Appellate Division reversed the convictions in all three cases. The *Onofre* Court, extending the right of privacy to consenting adults, invalidated the law prohibiting consensual sodomy and extended to individuals the protected right to engage in homosexual acts and in all heterosexual contacts. It used prior decisions regarding birth control [24], abortion [38], and the right to read obscene material in one's home [43] and extended that right of privacy developed in those cases to the right to choose one's *means* of sexual gratification.

Applying the doctrine of strict scrutiny (which must be applied to any state attempt to burden or restrict a fundamental right), and assessing the ability of the state to demonstrate harm, the *Onofre* Court declared that the state lacked the power, in the absence of a showing of a clear harm, to criminalize the conduct. It declared this despite the fact that a legislative majority had deemed such behavior immoral. It found personal sexual conduct to be a fundamental right "protected by the right to privacy because of the transcendental importance of sex to the human condition, the intimacy of conduct, and its relationship to a person's right to control his or her own body" [30]. Thus the court extended the right of privacy to the means of sexual gratification creating a logically coherent doctrine. The court stated that one has a right "to make decisions with respect to the consequence of sexual encounters and, necessarily, to have such encounters" [31]. It concluded that within areas of sexuality and individual rights, the state had demonstrated no harm, either physical harm to the participant or harm to the public morality, and that therefore there was "no rational basis . . . for excluding from the same protection decisions to seek sexual gratification from what was once commonly regarded as deviant conduct" [31].

Onofre argues that the equal protection clause permitted no rational distinction (as *Eisenstadt v. Baird* [21] had established) between married and unmarried persons, and thus should, by extension, permit no distinction between heterosexuals or homosexuals. It further commented that there was no "rational basis upon which the Legislature could have decided to freely allow the conduct in issue among married people and to make identical conduct criminal among those for whom that state is undesirable or unattainable" [31]. *Onofre* established a fundamental right which includes a "generalized right to gratification in whatever form it should be" [31]. The right gives unlimited choice of the

means of sexual satisfaction as long as these are choices made voluntarily by adults in non-commercial, private, non-public settings [31].
The case establishes that in areas of fundamentally guarded sexuality,
criminal laws are inappropriate unless the state can produce clear
empirical evidence of harm.

People v. Onofre fashions a realm of protected sexual expression from
a doctrine of protected procreational choice. As with cases empowering
persons to refuse medical treatment and defy paternalism, it prohibits
the sort of paternalism practiced by legislatures, in enacting statutes
based on majoritarian moralism without a demonstration of compelling
state interest. *Onofre* establishes the principle that generally understood
concepts of sexual morality no longer have legal sanction readily available.

The case establishes a right to sexual satisfaction, sexual preference,
free sexual expression and sexual gratification. It protects the process
rather than the end result of a sexual liaison as the earlier cases did. It
raises some fascinating questions however. If there is a fundamental
right to sexual gratification between consenting adults, is there some
obligation on the part of the state, in certain circumstances, to provide
the means or at least the space for the expression of that right?

Consider, for example, the plight of the institutionalized, be they
mentally ill, mentally retarded, persons in nursing homes, or persons
convicted of crimes. For this last category of persons there is an
argument that effective care and custody required by jailing and the
punishment permitted in prisons would not require that the state provide the opportunity for sexual expression. The demise of the "least
restrictive alternative" doctrine [45] in regard to jailed inmates and the
reaffirmation of necessities of prison administration would most probably preclude the argument. However, even for prison inmates, given a
fundamental right to sexual gratification, given the state obligation to
avoid "deliberate indifference to serious medical needs of prisoners"
[22], and given the inextricable link between sexuality and mental
health, the argument is not unforseeable.

There is a more compelling, less forceful and more immediate set of
arguments, however, in regard to the rights of sexual expression and
gratification for those in mental institutions and in nursing homes. This
argument is buttressed by another line of cases interpreting the 'right to
privacy.' Two cases, *Rennie v. Klein* [37] and *Okin v. Rogers* [28] (*sub
nom Mills v. Rogers* in the Supreme Court [27]) have established, at

least in the first and second circuit, that there is a qualified right to refuse psychotropic medications, which applies not only to those voluntarily committed to mental institutions but to the involuntarily committed as well. This right to refuse is based upon interpretations of the right to privacy and is dependent upon, in some measure, the judgment that decision-making capabilities of the mentally ill may in fact be appropriate to the decision to refuse treatment, which is protected by the constitution.

If the mentally ill and the confined have the constitutionally protected right to refuse psychotropic medications, deemed in their best interests, would they not, at least in New York, have the right to the further expression of their guaranteed privacy interests through the ability to act in fulfillment of sexual needs and preferences? The concept may conjure up the image of people of limited or diminished capacity expressing sexual preference in ways unpleasant or unappetizing or perverted. That, however, may be more a reflection of the prejudice of us, the non-institutionalized, than the reality of the situation. Those confined in state institutions for treatment are clearly not stripped of their constitutional rights; most are legally competent. Sexual expression, if protected, should also be protected for these persons.

Consider also the issue of nursing homes. The regimentation in these institutions is no less restrictive than that in many mental institutions or indeed in more benevolent prisons. Sexuality between inhabitants is often severely punished. Onanism is puritanically decreed. It is forbidden for doors to be locked, for quiet corners to be occupied, for touching to occur. Would it be unreasonable for nursing homes to provide the needed space for sexuality? Perhaps they cannot provide single rooms for all of their inhabitants; but what of quiet and private rooms where two people could go to be alone? Would that not be a proper subject for state regulation? If people have rights, others may be required to assist in the exercise of those rights, especially in total institutions.

If there is a right to sexual gratification, there is no logical barrier to extending this right to the mentally ill and the mentally retarded. The state or institution must then refrain from interfering with the exercise of that right, and may be required to provide adequate opportunity. The *Onofre* case, however, couched its language only as relevant to consenting adults. Can the mentally ill or the old of diminished capacities be so classified? Quite clearly, yes. This argument is supported both if the people are competent and even, in a perverse way, if incompetent.

Over the last two decades, majoritarian, Victorian morality has disintegrated in the face of popular culture. The one area in which it is possible for the state to enforce this morality is over those it confines or controls directly in state institutions or correctional centers, or indirectly in nursing homes. Many of these people are no less able to be aroused sexually [2], no less able to receive sexual gratification, and no less protected by the right of privacy.

The *Onofre* case, however, raises the question of whether there is any legitimate interest of the state in how people use or abuse their bodies. Should the state care how individual preference is expressed? How direct and immediate must be the showing of harm? What evidence will suffice? What dire consequences must occur before the state is again permitted to establish the norms for behavior? Is individual decision-making the only permissible rule?

Consider, for example, the epidemic development of Acquired-Immune Deficiency Syndrome (AIDS). AIDS is presently posing a possible sex-related epidemic of justifiable concern. To date, according to the National Center for Disease Control, more than 3,600 cases of AIDS have been reported [3], with many more in the probable category. Of these, over 1,500 have died, and there is no reasonable expectation that any will survive [3]. Theories of transmission include passing by intimate personal contact or by the mixing of body secretions. One hypothesis is that this disease is transmitted by some sort of infectious agent such as exists in hepatitis. The probability, given the pattern of infection, is that of an infectious agent passed most directly through bodily products such as saliva, urine, semen, stool and sweat. The persons most likely to contract the disease are homosexuals, Haitians, hemophiliacs and I.V. drug users [1].

Persons who have AIDS experience periodic admissions to hospitals for treatment of infections which their bodies cannot combat. During their hospital stay they are kept in isolation. Special care is taken with their body secretions; blood is specially labelled; all body products are transported in plastic bags; laboratories are alerted to use special gloves and procedures. When the acute stage has passed, however, the person is released into the community.

In between periodic hospitalization, persons with AIDS are released into the community to live with families, to exercise their sexual prefer-

ence and to satisfy sexual appetites. One physician discharging a homosexual AIDS patient back to the community to live with his parents and
younger siblings and to roam the gay community, anguished over his
inability to prevent a pattern of behavior which he feared might lead to
the spread of the disease. Epidemiological evidence thus far demonstrates clusters of the disease often linked to one person. He begged his
patient not to go back on the fast track of indiscriminate sexual liaisons.
He knew that the dreaded pattern would most likely be re-established.

Should the law have some power to regulate the course of conduct of
these persons between hospital admissions? Individual contract law is of
course always an option. Consent to sexual contact would be vitiated by
fraud. Non-revelation of AIDS could be held to invalidate the consent
of an adult and may support a suit for money damages brought by the
unknowing partner. This, however, offers little comfort for the possibly
infected.

How clear, concrete and direct must be the evidence of transmiss-
ibility before harm to the public is demonstrated and state interest
established? Attempts have been made to exclude homosexuals from
blood bank collections for fear that they are AIDS-infected or hepatitis-
infected [3]. Is this an acceptable request by the public or demand by the
state? Is it constitutional? Must patterns reach epidemic proportions
before a state may exercise a legitimate interest in protecting the public
health?

Consider the epidemic of herpes virus – which some construe as the
revenge of biology on recreational sex. Modern methods of contraception have ensured that sexual acts can be performed almost without
procreational consequences. Yet Herpes demonstrates that recreational
sex can have other consequences. Herpes, if undiagnosed, unrecognized
and untreated, may have terrible consequences for a fetus [5]. May it
have other consequences? When these are discovered, will there be
some calculus which is constitutionally legitimate and which permits the
state to reassert its interest in the protection of the public by the
prohibition of certain very personal actions?

Underlying these questions is of course a concern for the consequence
not only for the individual but for the state. A major problem presented
by sodomy laws and other sorts of statutes which attempt to interfere
with private consenting behavior is the impossibility of adequate
enforcement [24]. Were we to make new laws restricting individual

action, would we be willing to enforce them? And if the enforcement is either impossible, or if possible, with such damage to the fabric of the state to be infeasible, then is prohibition reasonable?

American society has reached a point of individual preference in matters of sexuality and the control of procreation. There is a right to control reproduction, a right to procreate, and one could argue by extension of these, a pendant, though not protected, right to fornicate; the chaos in the law does not clearly support this extension. The questions for society are yet to be posed. This exclusive focus on the individual and the necessity that the state demonstrate a compelling interest supported by weighty evidence to infringe individual rights, has permitted the deification of patterns of behavior which previous cultures labelled morally decadent.

Is there in fact no societal stake in the sexual coupling and uncoupling of its citizens? Is there no relationship between sexuality and the patterns of family stability or instability? Is the breakdown of the nuclear family destructive to society? Is that related to patterns of recreational sex? How would one go about assessing this dimension of harm and weighing such harm to society against the clear infringement of individual right and the unseemly exercise of police power which the criminalization of private conduct must entail? Such will be some of the issues for the next decade.

Montefiore Medical Center
The Bronx, New York City

ACKNOWLEDGMENT

Research and editorial assistance were kindly provided by· Connie Zuckerman.

BIBLIOGRAPHY

1. Altman, L.: Jan. 5, 1984, 'New Cases Widen Views About AIDS', *The Times, New York*, A-20 col. 1.
2. Brecher, E.: *Love, Sex and Aging*, Little, Brown and Co., Boston, Mass.
3. Chase, M.: March 12, 1984, 'Gift of Love May also Be an Agent of Death in Some AIDS Cases', *Wall Street Journal*, p. 1, col. 1.
4. Grosboll, D.: 1980, 'Sterilization Abuse: Current State of the Law and Remedies for Abuse', *Golden Gate University Law Review* **10**, 1147.

5. Hamilton, R.: 1980, *The Herpes Book*, J. P. Tarcher, Los Angeles, Calif.
6. Holmes, O. W.: 1881, *The Common Law*, Little, Brown and Co., Boston, Mass.
7. Holmes, O. W.: 1920, 'The Path of the Law', *Collected Legal Papers*, Harcourt, Brace and Howe, New York, N.Y.
8. Kinsey, A., Pameroy, W., and Martin, C.: 1948, *Sexual Behavior in the Human Male*, W. B. Saunders Co., Philadelphia, Penn.
9. Marmor, J. (ed.),: 1980, *Homosexual Behavior*, Basic Books, New York, N.Y.
10. *New York City Administration Code*, Section 22, Title C, 1977.
11. Novak, J., Rotunda, R., and Young, J.: 1983, *Constitutional Law*, West Publishing Co., St. Paul, Minn.
12. *Oxford English Dictionary*, 1901, Clarendon Press, Oxford, U.K.
13. Prosser, W.: 1971, *The Law of Torts*, West Publishing Co., St. Paul, Minn.
14. Rivera, R.: 1979, 'Our Straight-Laced Judges: The Legal Position of Homosexual Persons in the United States,' *Hastings Law Journal* **30**, 799.
15. *Akron v. Akron Center For Reproductive Health Inc.*, 103 S. Ct. 2481, 1983.
16. *Buck v. Bell*, 274 U.S. 200, 1927.
17. *Canterbury v. Spence*, 464 F.2d 772, D.C. Cir., 1972.
18. *Carey v. Population Serv. Int.'l*, 431 U.S. 678, 1977.
19. *Cobbs v. Grant*, 502 P.2d 1, CA, 1972.
20. *Doe v. Commonwealth's Attorney* 403 F. Supp. 1199, VA, 1975.
21. *Eisenstadt v. Baird*, 405 U.S. 438, 1972.
22. *Estelle V. Gamble*, 429 U.S. 97, 1976.
23. *In re Grady*, 405 A.2d 851, NJ, 1979.
24. *Griswold v. Connecticut*, 381 U.S. 479, 1965.
25. *Hathaway v. Worcester City Hospital*, 475 F.2d 701, 1st Cir., 1973.
26. *Lane v. Candura*, 376 N.E. 2d 1232, MA, 1978.
27. *Mills v. Rogers*, 102 S.Ct. 2442, 1982.
28. *Okin v. Rogers*, 634 F.2d 650, 1st Cir., 1980.
29. *Olmstead v. United States*, 277 U.S. 438, 1928.
30. *People v. Onofre*, 424, N.Y.S.2d 566, 1980.
31. *People v. Onofre*, 434 N.Y.S.2d 947, 1980.
32. *Planned Parenthood of Missouri v. Danforth*, 428 U.S. 52, 1976.
33. *In re President and Directors of Georgetown College*, 331 F.2d 1000, D.C. Cir., 1978.
34. *In re Quackenbush*, 383 A.2d 785, NJ, 1978.
35. *In re Quinlan*, 355 A.2d 647, NJ, 1976.
36. *Relf v. Weinberger*, 372 F.Supp. 1196, D.C. Cir., 1974.
37. *Rennie v. Klein*, 653, F.2d 836, 3rd Cir., 1981.
38. *Roe v. Wade*, 410 U.S. 113, 1973.
39. *Ruby v. Massey*, 452 F.Supp. 361, CT, 1978.
40. *Satz v. Perlmutter*, 379 So.2d 359, FL, 1980.
41. *Schloendorff v. Society of N.Y. Hosp.*, 105 N.E. 92, NY, 1914.
42. *Skinner v. Oklahoma*, 316 U.S. 535, 1942.
43. *Stanley v. Georgia*, 394 U.S. 557, 1969.
44. *Superintendent of Belchertown State School v. Saikewicz*, 370 N.E.2d 417, MA, 1977.
45. *Wolfish v. Levi*, 573, F.2d 118, 2nd Cir., 1978.
46. *In re Yetter*, 62 Pa.D. & C.2d 619, 1973.

CONSTANCE A. NATHANSON

FAMILY PLANNING AND CONTRACEPTIVE RESPONSIBILITY

INTRODUCTION

In an address to the National Association of Evangelicals on March 8, 1983, President Reagan made the following comments in reference to the federal government's attempt to require parental notification when contraceptives are prescribed to teenagers 17 and under:

Girls termed 'sexually active' – that has replaced the word 'promiscuous' – are given 'birth control drugs and devices' by federally subsidized clinics in order to prevent illegitimate birth or abortion. In discussions of this issue no one seems to mention morality as playing a part in the subject of sex. Is all of Judeo-Christian tradition wrong? Are we to believe that something so sacred can be looked upon as a purely physical thing with no potential for emotional and psychological harm? And isn't it the parents' right to give counsel and advice to keep their children from making mistakes that may affect entire lives? . . . The rights of parents and the rights of family take precedence over those of Washington-based bureaucrats and social engineers (*New York Times*, March 9, 1983).

These remarks may best be understood as one more salvo in a battle over the meaning and management of sexual behavior that, at least in its more public manifestations, has been going on in American society since the middle of the nineteenth century: Who has the right to define the meaning of sexual behavior? Who has the right to control this behavior? Who is responsible for the consequences of sexual behavior? Alignment in this struggle is clearly reflected in the way words are used: 'Promiscuous', for example, suggests a quite different approach to issues of responsibility and control than does 'sexually active', as the President, no doubt, intended. The President is at pains to speak of "birth control drugs and devices" rather than to use the more respectable euphemism, 'family planning', a term adopted by the leaders of the birth control movement in 1942 on the advice of a public relations consultant. The President, we may be sure, has his own consultants. Finally, the President poses the issue of control very clearly, as between organized clinics supported by "Washington-based bureaucrats" and the family supported, implicitly, by the church.

Contraception for married women is no longer a moral issue for most Americans. For reasons to be amplified below, the field of battle has

183

Stuart F. Spicker, William B. Bondeson, and H. Tristram Engelhardt, Jr.
The Contraceptive Ethos, 183–197.
© 1987 *by D. Reidel Publishing Company.*

shifted to contraception for unmarried teenage girls. Nevetheless, the basic arguments over morality and responsibility remain unchanged. The purpose of this paper is not to advocate a particular position in the struggle to which I allude (although I will state my own position in order to avoid ambiguity). It is, rather, to clarify the major questions that surround the issue of contraceptive responsibility as they appear from the perspective of individuals directly involved in providing contraceptive services to unmarried young women. One of the consequenses of the way in which contraceptive technology has been developed in this country, a consequence that is quite clearly contested in President Reagan's remarks, is that responsibility for provision of contraceptive services has devolved upon the medical profession. Reagan's comments about 'Washington-based bureaucrats' and 'social engineers' notwithstanding, this responsibility is a considerable source of discomfort for those who are constrained to exercise it. To identify the sources of that discomfort is to shed light on some of the basic dilemmas that are raised by the availability of effective contraception.

A PERSONAL DIGRESSION

My own position on the issue of contraceptive responsibility is very simply stated, although I will present one or two arguments in its favor. By making contraception available to women (and I refer to all women of reproductive age irrespective of age or marital status), we neither condone vice nor impose virtue. We merely provide women who are engaging in sexual intercourse with the means of preventing unwanted pregnancy. Morally or ethically, the use of contraception is not different from the use of seat belts; it represents a reasonable precaution against a known risk. To impose conditions on the accessibility or use of contraception makes no more sense than to impose conditions on the accessibility or use of seat belts. Unfortunately, in our society, conditions are most likely to be imposed on, or experienced by, the very individuals most prone to accidents, namely young unmarried women. Indeed, just as a more mature adult might advise a youngster to put on his or her seat belt, so adults should advise children on the use of contraception. Not to do so, on the grounds that individuals under a certain age should not be taking these risks in the first place, is an abdication of adult responsibility.

In addition, the existence of effective contraception does not imply any moral obligation that it be used, Use or non-use are matters of individual choice, with the provisos that choice should be as informed as possible and that individuals should be assisted to avoid the consequences of contraceptive mistakes rather than be punished for them.

I will propose to slip back into my role as a sociologist and use my own research on contraceptive services for teenagers as the basis for an analysis of the social control of sexual behavior as performed in county health department family planning clinics. However, at the conclusion of this paper, I will return to the more general issues that I have raised.

SOCIAL CONTROL OF SEXUAL BEHAVIOR: CONTRACEPTIVE SERVICES FOR TEENAGERS

The Clinic Setting

County Health Department Family Planning Clinics are the major organized sources of birth control services for teenagers. Approximately 20% of young women under 20 obtain their method – usually the pill – from a local Health Department Clinic. Picture a one story red brick building, surrounded by a small plot of poorly tended grass, and a large expanse of asphalt, populated by no-longer-new, government issue sedans in unobtrusive colors. Walk up the few steps into a large, open waiting room, benches aligned in meeting-house fashion as if waiting for the service to begin. On the walls are posters, often handmade, extolling the virtues of good nutrition (with vivid, if inexpert, illustrations of apples and cheese), the evils of cigarettes and alcohol, or, one of my favorites, displaying baby pictures from the clinic's former maternity patients. On a typical family planning clinic morning at a busy clinic, the waiting room pews are fully occupied by lank-haired young women, and a few men, all identically attired in blue jeans, sitting in rows to face the invisible minister. The silence of the waiting patients is broken by the yelling of babies, the shushing of tired and impatient mothers – "I'm going to whip you!' – muttered under the breath, and, like a baseball commentator announcing the batting order, the periodic appearance from somewhere backstage of a clinic nurse, neatly clad in inevitable blue, calling the next patient.

Although the foregoing description is reasonably typical, clinics can vary tremendously in atmosphere, from rushed, harassed and harassing, to cheerful and relaxed, depending on the size of the premises, the number of patients waiting to be seen, the number of staff available to see them, and on the manner in which that staff goes about its business. The basic elements of clinic procedure are, however, remarkably unvarying across the 78 clinics we studied; these procedures are based on guidelines established by the State Health Department Family Planning Division. From the perspective of this paper, the most important component of these procedures are the contraceptive education and counseling sessions. Always conducted by a clinic nurse, it is through these sessions that the nurses convey to the clients *their* contraceptive philosophy.

In the context of Health Department Family Planning Clinics, birth control pills (and other contraceptive methods, although pills are far and away the most popular method in these clinics) are not a morally neutral technology for preventing unwanted pregnancy, to be dispensed over the counter like aspirin or Vitamin C, but a vehicle for teaching personal and moral responsibility. This orientation is best reflected in the question put to me by a nursing director with whom I was chatting informally: "Are we teaching responsibility if we call a patient when she misses an appointment?" One may question the consistency of this concern with the clinic's overt objective of providing contraceptive protection, but it is quite consistent with the more covert character-building objectives to which I have referred.

In a darkened room, four or five black teenagers sit quietly watching an educational film depicting a white girl talking to a white nurse about contraception. The real-live white nurse who will run today's educational session has not yet arrived and the noise of the ancient 16 millimeter movie projector effectively drowns out the soundtrack, limiting the film to a purely visual message. Suddenly lights are switched on, a brisk young woman in blue walks in and takes up her position in front of today's class. Contraceptive education is about to begin.

Although the format varies across clinics, the content of these educational sessions remains the same, following health department guidelines. Included are sexual anatomy and physiology, a review of clinic procedures, and a discussion of alternative contraceptive methods. This content is the medium through which the clinic's message of responsibility, autonomy and good morals is transmitted.

The first part of the session is over. A poll of the young clients quickly establishes that the pill is their unanimous choice of contraceptive method. The nurse will focus on the pill, going over the other methods, as she says, 'lightly'. Turning to the pill, she begins, "they only work if you take them right. Our job is to make sure that you take them right'. Taking them 'right' the clients find, imposes conformity to a complex and detailed set of rules and procedures, regulating the most intimate details of conduct. This is how it goes:

You must start your pills on the Sunday after the first day of your next menstrual period, ("this way," the nurse jokes, "you will never have your period on a weekend," setting off a wave of giggles), "you must use foam and condoms with your entire first pack of pills (and it would be better if you don't have sex for the first ten pills); you must use foam and condoms if you miss even one pill; if you miss three, you must use foam and condoms till the end of the pack. You must take the pill at the same time every day. You must always remember the type of pill you've been taking and the date of your last menstrual period. Finally, you must never say, 'I got pregnant because I lost my pills.'

As this latter comment suggests, the ever-present implication is that failure to conform with the clinic-prescribed regimen will result in pregnancy. The new 'good girl' may be 'sexually active', but she takes her pills by the book. This shift in the focus of normative attention from chastity to compliance is not lost on clients; they fully expect that conformity to procedural requirements will result in protection against pregnancy, and are correspondingly disturbed when problems arise, as exemplified by the following comments from a young clinic patient:

I've had no period for three months, I did everything by the rule book. Some girls in my high school don't care – they get pregnant. I did everything carefully. It isn't normal that I shouldn't have my period. I do everything right. I'm not a bad girl.

In a classic shift in the 'paradigm of deviance designation' [10], 'sin' has been redefined from having sex outside of marriage to having sex outside the rules for contraceptive protection. The 'wages of sin' are still unwanted pregnancy, but the arbiters of 'sinful' behavior are no longer theologians but physicians and nurses. This paradigm shift is exactly what President Reagan attacks in his remarks, cited earlier.

As Schneider and Conrad note in their extremely useful analysis of the medicalization of deviant behavior [10], changes in designations of deviance carry in their train changes in 'reality' as well as rhetoric. Among the consequences of defining the prevention of unwanted pregnancy as a medical rather than a moral problem are changes in the appropriate agents of social control from moral to medical authorities (a change strongly contested in Reagan's remarks), changes in the meaning of the behavior in question (from 'promiscuity' to 'sexual activity'), changes in the arena where deviance is identified (from the home, the courts, or the pulpit to the family planning clinic), and changes in the mode of intervention (from the threat of pregnancy at the worst, to lasting social ostracism, à la 'The French Lieutenant's Woman at the best, to the pill). That the medical profession has a more than trivial investment in protecting its jurisdiction over the control of unwanted pregnancy against encroachment by the advocates of traditional morality is indicated by the line-up of every major national medical and public health organization in opposition to the Reagan administration's parental notification rule.

Notwithstanding this evidence of organizational solidarity in the face of external threat, ownership of the turf represented by teenage pregnancy creates profound dilemmas for medical professionals, and particularly for physicians and nurses with direct service responsibilities – the front-line of unwanted pregnancy control. It is through a description and analysis of these dilemmas that the question of contraceptive responsibility can be addressed. The personal and professional orientations of family planning nurses (nurses are the key figures in health department clinics and will be the principal focus of this discussion) cause them to approach the provision of contraceptive services to teenagers with marked ambivalence; this ambivalence is resolved by structuring the encounter between provider and client so as to maximize the client's responsibility for contraceptive decisions and outcomes and to minimize that of the provider. I introduce my analysis with a brief description of the background and attitudinal orientations that nurses bring to their clinic work and an even more succinct account of that work itself.

The Nurse

The average family planning clinic nurse is a 42 year old married woman with two or three children, who has worked in the county health department for six years. However, both age and length of service cover a wide range. The oldest nurse with whom we spoke was 71, the youngest, 25; 21% of the nurses have been in their county health department jobs for 13 years or more. About two-thirds of the nurses are Protestant, 27% Catholic; only 15 out of 376 professed 'no religion'. Of more significance, 75% stated that religion was at least 'moderately' important in their lives; 49% that it was 'very important'. Finally, and most importantly, as a group these women have very traditional attitudes toward premarital sex. Only 24% approve of an unmarried girl having sex with a boy with whom she is in love; less than half approve even if marriage is intended. The implications of these attitudes for the structuring of the nurses' family planning clinic role are considered below.

As a basis for understanding the nurse's orientation to her clinic role, it is also important to be aware that few nurses have chosen to work in the family planning clinic. It is simply one aspect of their assignment as county health department staff nurses. Over 90% work in other clinics as well, and, indeed, 54% *prefer* to work in other clinics (only 24% prefer family planning; the rest state no preference).

The principal work of the clinic nurse is patient interviewing and counselling; nurses also do the blood work that is required for family planning clinic patients, take blood pressures, and are present during the physical examination by the physician. Although the focus of this paper is on teenagers, all but six of the 78 clinics we studied see women of all age groups combined. As a final note, before proceeding to a broader analysis of the nurse's role, we asked nurses which age group they found *easier* to work with and which one they *preferred* to work with. Among the nurses willing to state a preference, only 24% found teens easier to work with than older women but, in testimony to their readiness for challenge, 62% preferred to work with teens.

The Nurse's Clinic Role

The role of the nurse in the family planning clinic is a particularly difficult one. These difficulties are, in part, generic to the role of the professional with a lay clientele, and include problems of obtaining recognition of professional authority and compliance with professional advice [1]. However, these generic problems are compounded in the present case by characteristics peculiar to the 'condition' for which 'treatment' in the family planning clinic is sought and by the nature of the treatment itself.

Attribution of responsibility is a central issue in determining societal responses to deviant behavior. The reaction to a violation of social norms will, as Freidson points out, be very different depending on whether the cause "is seen to lie in deliberate choice rather than in accident, inheritance, infection, or witchcraft" ([2], p. 334). Conditions for which the individual is held responsible tend to be treated punitively while involuntary conditions are managed with permissive treatment or instruction. Sexual intercourse, for which the appropriate treatment is birth control if pregnancy is unwanted, is inherently ambiguous with respect to questions both of deviance and responsibility. In itself it is neither deviant nor irresponsible. Whether or not intercourse is socially *defined* as deviant or irresponsible depends entirely on the conditions under which it occurs. And how intercourse is socially defined determines how the 'treatment' for intercourse is regarded. Thus, Margaret Sanger in her campaign to 'sell' birth control to medical and social elites was at pains to portray the potential clients for this service as poor, hard-working married women, more often than not the victims of an insatiable husband, consequently neither deviant nor irresponsible [8]. By contrast, Reagan, in advocating the parental notification rule, focuses entirely on the deviance of the behavior in question: sexual intercourse by unmarried girls "below the age of consent" transgresses moral norms and should, therefore, receive moral, not medical, treatment.

In their encounters with teenage clients, family planning nurses find themselves in a most uncomfortable position with respect to these issues of deviance and responsibility. By background and orientation, these nurses are conventional women with highly traditional moral values. By virtue of their positions as health department employees they are, nevertheless, socially mandated (a mandate hotly contested, of course, in the public policy arena) to provide an essentially medical, that is, non-punitive service directed toward preventing young women from experiencing the consequences of what many nurses regard as their immoral behavior. Reconciliation of this conflict is accomplished by redefining virtue as contraceptive 'responsibility', that is, conformity to a set of detailed rules and procedures for contraceptive use, (and for other aspects of client behavior as well), and by heavily emphasizing the pedagogical as opposed to the dispensary functions of the family planning nurse. As one of the nurse commented, "it's very nice to be able to say to parents, 'she's got to go to a group, we don't dispense pills like candy'." By structuring their role in terms of character-building, nurses are able to sustain a satisfying professional self-image, despite their profound ambivalence towards the behavior that creates the need for their services. There are, nevertheless, certain inherent contradictions in this role if the functions of a family planning clinic are defined as assisting women to prevent unwanted pregnancy rather than as contributing to the develoment of moral responsibility. These contradictions and the conflicts which they engender may be illustrated by an examination of nurses' conceptions of the desirable, as contrasted with the undesirable, teenage client.

Complementing the nurse's conception of her role as educator and counselor, the most rewarding client is the one who is eager to learn: "knows what you've been talking about and absorbs the 'instructions', interested in learning something about herself". The girl who 'is interested', and 'asks questions and responds' is, furthermore, the one who is perceived as a potentially good contraceptor. Similarly, the undesirable client is the one who is perceived as disinterested in, or actively rejecting of the educational/counseling component of the nurses' role: "the ones who sit and just want the pill and not the advice that goes with it", who say "just give me pills and don't ask a lot of questions". Girls with this orientation are a problem for the nurse on two levels: first, they undermine the very foundations of professional authority by not only prescribing for themselves but attempting to set the terms on which the prescription is received; second, they reject what is, to the family planning nurse, the most-valued component of her professional role by treating her as an 'over-the-counter' pill dispenser. In these circumstances, the weight of the health department bureaucracy is, of course, all on the side of the nurse: education and counseling (as well as history-taking, blood work, and a complete physical examination) are conditions (and 78% of the nurses 'strongly agree' that they should be conditions) for receiving a birth control method. Furthermore, nurses believe that teenage clients who do not show interest in the educational sessions are unlikely to be good contraceptors. Whether they are right or wrong, the potential for conflict with clients who have a different service model in mind should be clear.

A second major dimension of client 'desirability,' conformity to clinic procedures, is a direct consequence of the somewhat formalistic, even ritualistic, content of education and counseling in family planning clinics, and of the inherently bureaucratic nature of the clinics themselves. Earlier, the rules for 'correct' pill-taking were described. The salience of procedural issues in structuring client-provider interaction is further enhanced by clinic practice of: (1) giving out only three packs of pills at the first visit, and (2) requiring a complete annual physical examination to renew the pill prescription. In addition, fewer than half of the clinics accept clients without a scheduled appointment even 'occasionally' and less than a third hold evening or Saturday hours. In these circumstances, opportunities abound for teenage clients to miss appointments, run out of pills, request emergency visits at unscheduled times, and the like. Between the complexities of the contraceptive regimen and of the clinic's procedures, it is perhaps not surprising that nurses are highly sensitive to the question of who is 'at fault' if a pregnancy occurs. This issue will be returned to later in the paper.

The rewarding client, then, is the one who conforms – who keeps her appointments and uses her method correctly. The term 'responsibility' is constantly on the lips of clinic nurses, and one (among several) of its meanings is conformity to clinic and contraceptive rules. Similarly, the 'irresponsible' client is the one who does not follow the rules: she "comes back pregnant because she doesn't bother to follow instructions". She will say, "I only skipped one pill and look what happend", or she will "call and say, 'I'm out of pills'", and want to come in right away instead of at scheduled clinic time.

Underlying these conceptions of the desirable patient is the nurses' struggle to control the sexual and contraceptive behavior of their teenage clients, a struggle which reflects their ambivalence toward the behavior itself. Control is exercised in two partially contradictory ways: first, through education and counseling, consisting of detailed prescriptions for having 'responsible' sex, and second, through clinic procedural requirements. The principal sanction against non-conformity to the former set of rules is the threat of pregnancy: "the pills won't work if you don't take them right". The major sanction against non-conformity to clinic administrative procedures is the threat of being unable to obtain the pills. Lapses in conformity to either set of rules are attributed to client 'irresponsibility.' Given that nurses use their position as gatekeepers (their control over access to resources desired by the client) to insist that contraception is obtained on *their terms*, this conception of the 'irresponsible' client seems virtually inevitable. Otherwise, pregnancy could conceivably be blamed on the barriers that prevent the client from getting contraception on *her* terms, an issue to which nurses are quite sensitive. Correct use of oral contraception *does* require adherence to a scheduled routine, and organizations *do* need certain rules to facilitate the orderly conduct of their business. However, reliance on a detailed set of rules and procedures also functions, at least in part, to absolve the nurse of responsibility for 'mistakes'.

Earlier, it was noted that 'responsibility' in family planning clinic parlance, means conformity to clinic procedures. It is also used to mean autonomy. The desirable patient, the girl who is perceived to be a potentially good contraceptor, makes her decision to attend the clinic free of any external influence – "if mother (or boyfriend or girlfriends) made her come, she won't be a good contraceptor". She makes an independent choice of contraceptive method – "we try hard not to be trapped into recommending a method". Finally, of course, she adheres to the method and does not blame the clinic when things go wrong. (There is a striking aversion among clinic staff to 'follow-up' of clients after they have left the clinic, an aversion which is justified by reference to the need to inculcate 'responsibility' by discouraging dependency.)

The ideology of client autonomy, like the heavy reliance on procedural details, serves, in part, to protect the nurse from feeling responsible if a client 'comes back pregnant'. However, the inherently contradictory nature of nurses' expectations for client behavior is readily apparent. The 'independent' autonomous client who comes to the clinic knowing what she wants is correspondingly less likely to be uncritically accepting of clinic procedures. The client who is less sure of herself, on the other hand, may readily accept what the clinic has to offer, but have great difficulty in making autonomous contraceptive decisions. Clients in the latter mold are potentially the most vulnerable to nurses' preference for character-building over pregnancy-prevention.

This analysis of the role of the family planning nurse has shown how individuals directly involved in the provision of contraceptive services to a morally suspect set of clients resolve conflicts between their personal moral orientations and their professional responsibilities. They do this in three ways: first, by redefining 'sin' from transgression of sexual norms to transgression of medical and bureaucratic norms; second, by structuring their professional role as one of developing personal and moral character; and, third, by absolving themselves, insofar as possible, from responsibility for failure. The latter point deserves brief elaboration. As Joffe [4] points out, "in family planning work, measures of 'success' are far more elusive than those of 'failure'". Feedback on contraceptive successes is rare; failure is all too visible. Furthermore, a teenage client who comes back to the clinic pregnant or after an abortion is a direct reminder of the underlying behavior for which contraception is the remedy. Her transgression of sexual norms is there for all to see; she is 'punished' by the presumption of responsibility for transgression of medical norms as well.

The Meaning of Contraceptive Responsibility

There are several reasons why the issue of responsibility may be particularly salient in the settings I have described. The age of the clientele –

in our study ranging from 11 through 19, with a median age of 16 –
renders nurses' expectations for an adult level of autonomous contraceptive complaince inherently problematic. 'Mistakes' are virtually
assured. Attribution of mistakes to client 'irresponsibility' arises only in
part from professional sensitivity to failure. At least two additional
motives appear to be at work. First, in claiming the turf represented by
adolescent pregnancy, the medical profession risks being held accountable for behavior it cannot fully control. The problematic nature of
control and, therefore, the size of the risk, are most apparent to workers
in direct contact with clients – 'street-level bureaucrats', to use Lipsky's
apt phraseology [6]. Concomitantly, it is at the 'street-level' that the need
to defend against this risk by stressing client responsibility – or irresponsibility, as the case may be – is most strongly felt. Second, behind the
fervor of nurses' condemnation lies the full weight of their underlying
disapproval of sexual behavior outside of marriage. By not condemning,
they may appear to condone not only lapses in contraceptive technique,
but lapses in personal morality as well.

Although questions concerning the meaning and locus of responsibility may be unusually prominent in the encounter between the family
planning nurse and her teenage client, they are by no means unique to
that setting. Attribution of responsibility to the client for following
medical direction (and corresponding condemnation for noncompliance, in which, as I. K. Zola notes [11], 'moral judgements [are] but a
pinprick below the surface''), are implicit in the medical model of social
control. The assumptions of the medical model are merely highlighted
and made more problematic when control is extended outside of the
consulting room and into the most intimate aspects of daily life. Problems very similar to those I have described between nurses and teenagers arise between genetic counselors and their clients [5, 7]. Clients
who, having been given full information about their risks of bearing an
affected child, state that they plan no more children but do nothing
about initiating effective contraception are a source of frustration to
genetic counselors; counselors' feelings closely resemble those of the
family planning nurse whose teenage client forgets her pills. From the
professional's perspective the client's behavior is irrational; behavior
that is perceived as irrational has a high probability of being labeled
irresponsible.

An extended analysis of the problem of 'drinking-driving', as Gusfield
calls it [3], describes the ways in which attributions of responsibility are

socially constructed. The problem of automobile safety and alcohol use is seen by concerned professionals as a problem of the individual motorist: drinking-driving is 'a choice by a willful person'. This perspective, Gusfield notes, tends to preclude attention to other aspects of the problem, for example, the role of "alcohol beverage distributors – bartenders, sellers, manufacturers" and of limitations in available modes of transportation during the hours and at the places where drinking is most likely to occur. Similarly, an exclusive focus on the 'willful' teenager may deflect attention from other possible loci of responsibility for teenagers' ineffective contraceptive use: the organizational structure of contraceptive services themselves, the inadequacies of available contraceptive methods, the ambivalence of adult society (including the families of sexually active adolescents) toward teenage sex, the circumstances under which teenagers have sex and use contraception, and the complex agendas of teenagers themselves.

To obtain at least one alternative perspective on the meaning of responsibility, it is only necessary to talk directly with young women concerning their experiences in using oral contraception. The pill is perceived as highly effective; however, not only does it have immediate side effects (side effects are the trigger for most pill discontinuations), but it is perceived as potentially dangerous both to the girl's own health and to the health of future offspring. Pill use, then, requires the continuous weighing of norms of responsible *contraceptive* protection against norms of responsible *health* protection. The boyfriend who urges our young woman to go off the pill in response to side effects may be perceived by clinic staff as encouraging irresponsibility, however, to the girl he is commendably more concerned about her health than about taking the rap for her pregnancy.

The danger that I perceive in family planning nurses' conception of responsibility (and, more generally, in the social construction of responsibility reflected in the medical model of deviance control) is, to quote Gusfield again, that "modes of conceiving of the reality of a phenomenon are closely related to the activities of resolution ([3], p. 6). Thus, the focus of family planning nurses on the shaping of responsible moral character appears to preclude certain activities that are logically related to the prevention of unwanted fertility, for example, the provision of active ongoing support to the novice contraceptive user in order to avoid contraceptive 'mistakes'. Reluctance to provide this support is justified on the grounds that coddling of clients will promote dependency; a more subtle implication is that individuals who are made to bear the consequences of their mistakes will learn to be more responsible. However, the cost of this lesson in responsibility is high if the consequence is unwanted pregnancy.

Much of this paper has been devoted to elucidating the origins of nurses' conceptions of responsibility, and I have argued above that their individualistic orientation blinds them to other ways of seeing the problem of teenage contraception and pregnancy and may inhibit a mere pluralistic approach to 'activities of resolution.' In closing, however, I will argue that it is possible to retain the conception of the responsible individual and, at the same time, to reject the corollary that responsibility must be reinforced by requiring individuals to bear the consequences of their mistakes. For my basic argument, I rely on the work of philosopher Janet Radcliffe Richards ([9], p. 223). Richards points out that,

There are in the nature of things no natural, inevitable consequences of most actions. People make mistakes and suffer setbacks as a result, but what happens in the long run depends not only on the nature of the mistake, but also on the action they take to put matters right afterwards . . . the only time when we insist that a particular consequence must follow a particular action . . . is *when the consequence is intended as a punishment.*

Unless pregnancy is deliberately intended as a punishment for contraceptive mistakes or for noncompliance with clinic rules, the only sensible course is to offer young women all possible assistance in avoiding both mistakes and their consequences; the younger and less mature the adolescent, the more assistance should be offered.

The Johns Hopkins University
Baltimore, Maryland

BIBLIOGRAPHY

1. Freidson, E.: 1965, 'The Impurity of Professional Authority', in H. S. Becker *et al.* (eds.), *Institutions and the Person*, Aldine, Chicago, Ill. pp. 25–34.
2. Freidson, E.: 1972, 'Disability as Social Deviance', in E. Freidson and J. Lorber (eds.), *Medical Men and Their Work*, Aldine, Chicago, Ill. pp. 330–52.
3. Gusfield, J. R.: 1981, *The Culture of Public Problems*, The University of Chicago Press, Chicago, Ill.
4. Joffe, C.: Unpublished manuscript.

5. Kessler, S.: 1980, 'The Psychological Paradigm Shift in Genetic Counseling', *Social Biology* **27**, 167–85.
6. Lipsky, M.: 1980, *Street-Level Bureaucracy*, Russell Sage, New York, NY.
7. President's Commission for the Study of Ethical Problems in Medicine and Biomedical and Behavioral Research 1983, *Screening and Counseling for Genetic Conditions*, U.S. Government Printing Office, Washington, D.C..
8. Reed, J.: 1978, *From Private Vice to Public Virtue: The Birth Control Movement and American Society Since 1830*, Basic Books, New York, NY.
9. Richards, J. R.: 1980, *The Skeptical Feminist*, Routledge and Kegan Paul, London, U.K..
10. Schneider, J. W. and Conrad, P.: 1980, 'The Medical Control of Deviance: Contests and Consequences', in J. Roth (ed.), *Research in the Sociology of Health Care*, Vol. I, JAI Press, Greenwich, Conn., pp. 1–53.
11. Zola, I. K.: 1975, 'Medicine as an Institution of Social Control', in C. Cox and A. Mead (eds.), *A Sociology of Medical Practice*, Collier-Macmillan, London, U.K., pp. 170–85.

WILLIAM B. BONDESON

PATIENT AUTONOMY, PATIENT CARE AND PROFESSIONAL RESPONSIBILITIES: THE HEALTH CARE PROFESSIONAL AS EDUCATOR AND PROVIDER OF SERVICES

Several of the contributors to this volume have made a claim which is central to a discussion of Professor Nathanson's paper; they have pointed out a kind of cultural consensus on the very absence of a cultural consensus. We do not agree, as a society, on the norms for reproductive or sexual activity. H. T. Engelhardt criticizes very ably in his paper the concept of the 'natural' in talking about sexual activity and sexual freedom, and he makes the case that there is no convincing and univocal definition of the term [2]. If, in the first place, we cannot make out a case for what is natural and what is not and, in the second place, if we are unable to generate any conclusive moral arguments as to what is acceptable or non-acceptable sexual behavior, then indeed we are in the very interesting position of trying to find ways to validate individual sexual preferences, however different they may be, only within the general limitations of some kind of harm to others. Within this boundary there do not seem to be any restrictions.

If it is wrong and inappropriate to create some kind of moral consensus by force, or coercion, or by the artificial creation of some kind of consensus through rational reconstruction such as some moral philosophers, for example Veatch [5], have tried to do, then we may be well advised to give up the attempt of trying to find some source of moral authority and instead decide to let people do what they think is best for themselves. But, of course, we really have not given up a source of moral authority at all, we have simply said that the source of moral authority is within each individual, acting by his or her own best likes and intentions. Individual freedom becomes the foundation for the moral authority of each individual. That moral authority of the individual then becomes the source of our social and legal principles, and it is inevitable that we will adopt different moral standards for ourselves insofar as we differ as human beings.

If one takes autonomy seriously as a right of self determination made possible by individual freedom, then there can also be a right to privacy

Stuart F. Spicker, William B. Bondeson, and H. Tristram Engelhardt, Jr.
The Contraceptive Ethos, 199–205.
© 1987 *by D. Reidel Publishing Company.*

which enables individuals to control the presentation of aspects of themselves to others. If the bodies of persons are indeed expressions of their personalities, and personalities are structures or hierarchies of values, then it follows that the use that is made of those bodies is just as much an expression of that person and personality as anything else. Thus, if we are to grant that privacy allows us to display and to form the self in all kinds of relationships with others, then sexual preferences are just another part of that hierarchy of relationships.

Contraceptive information and practices, within this context, allow for a greater freedom of sexual preference and activity because this information and these devices enable human beings to separate (a) the social aspects of sex insofar as relations are developed with other persons, (b) the recreational aspects of sex insofar as these are expressions of desire and attempts to gain pleasure for oneself, and (c) the reproductive aspects of sex insofar as these are attempts to create progeny. The separation of these aspects of sex and any others that there might be for that matter, is made possible, though neither guaranteed nor required, by the wide variety of contraceptive practices available in this country.

The moral issues to be considered here follow from the establishment of autonomy and privacy as conditions for the foundation and development of personhood and, once we have those conditions in place, then they make possible expressions of the self of all kinds, including sexual ones.

As Professor Dubler points out in her paper [1], if we begin with a right to sexual expression, and if we fail to make a persuasive distinction between 'natural' and 'unnatural' sexual practices, then such things as polygamy must be allowed if given the appropriate consent. If indeed we are to establish a right to sexual expression and sexual practices, then the only interesting moral questions which follow from that are not about the variety of sexual practices but rather about (a) who has the right (e.g., does it extend to the institutionalized in some form?), (b) who should serve as the sexual partner and are there any limitations on this activity, and (c) are there any limits to the kind of sexual activity to be allowed? I would suggest that if privacy and autonomy are taken as fundamental, then the only limitation that one might put on such sexual expression is demonstrable harm to others. But, there is much to be said as to the nature of this harm and its kinds. Physical, psychological and psychosocial harm all need to be delineated along with the concept of the risks of such harm. I cannot see an argument which limits, apart from this harm to others, the kinds of sexual activity in which one has the right to engage.

Professor Dubler very interestingly raises the point of such a right as applied to institutionalized persons and what kind of harm or risk of harm might be involved in such cases. There also needs to be a discussion of the age or level of competence of those who have the right to sexual expression.

One might look for limitations to this right in a kind of quasi-legal way by asking whether there are any interests of either the family or the state which might be affected by granting a right to sexual expression and activity. What might count as damage to an institution such as the family or the state is clearly a moral question, but whether or not granting certain rights to individuals actually brings about that kind of damage is an empirical question; there are at least four partly empirical questions Professor Nathanson's paper raises and which should be explored:

(1) Does the wide availability of contraceptive information and devices bring about an increase in sexual activity and in any particular kind of sexual activity?

(2) Does an increase in the availability of contraceptive information and devices lead to some kind of sexual exploitation (e.g., can this information be exploitative in a sub-culture which expects increased sexual activity on the part of its members because of the availability of this information and these devices)?

(3) Does an increase in the availability of contraceptive information and devices lead to a weakening, whatever that might mean, of the family, which in turn might somehow lead to a weakening of the moral fiber of state and society?

(4) Finally, does an increase in the availability of contraceptive information and practices lead to a greater sense of self-esteem and autonomy which helps people believe that they have some kind of greater control over their own bodies and their own destinies?

The above questions can only be answered by extensive research in the social sciences but on moral grounds it seems that we should do everything we can to increase the freedom and autonomy of individuals. As Janet Richards remarked most aptly, "The passion to decide to look after your fellow men, to do good to them in your way, is far more common than the desire to put into everyone's hand the power to look after themselves" [4].

Morally, we ought to put into everyone's hand the power to look after himself or herself and the question thus becomes: Does the increase in the availability of contraceptive information and devices lead to an increase in that autonomy, in that ability to look after oneself? I would guess that it does. But, of course, it will only work that way in the absence of countervailing pressures either from those who dispense this information or from a culture of fellow-users of that information which can be coercive.

Professor Nathanson, in addition to the above questions, raises some important moral issues about the roles and responsibilities of professions in general and, in particular, about the roles and responsibilities of the health professions. She points out that there has been a "shift in the paradigm of deviance designation" [3] from having sex outside of marriage to having sex outside the rules for contraceptive protection. I am not sure this is a real shift or is simply the addition of other roles and factors to the conception of what is sexually appropriate. She is right to point out that contraceptive information and methods have been medicalized to such an extent that the arbiters of what is right and wrong are no longer theologians but rather physicians and nurses.

It is also at least arguable whether or not the medical profession has a more than trivial investment in protecting its jurisdiction over the control of unwanted pregnancy against the encroachment of the advocates of traditional morality. I am not sure that this paradigm shift and the shift in the roles and responsibilities for monitoring, perhaps even worse, controlling sexual activity, is either a necessary or deliberate shift; society in many ways either tells or allows people in the medical profession to have the roles that they have. It is not necessarily the case that their adoption of these roles is of their own deliberate plan, choosing and campaign.

The ambivalence in the roles which health professionals can play moves between the role of educator and creator of autonomous, responsible people, and is another problem with Professor Nathanson's remarks. One of the ways to helpfully designate the roles and responsibilities of professions is to look at the relationship between professional and client as similar to the relationship between teacher and student. The role of the professional is understood, normatively that is, as an educational role, as having responsibilities to bring about that very freedom and autonomy, on the basis of information responsibly conveyed, that Professor Nathanson uses in her final quote from

Janet Richards. The philosophical issue is one which philosophers of education have been debating for years, namely whether education inescapably has normative and perhaps even propagandist aspects such that the attempt, via some kind of educational practice, to create personal autonomy, freedom and responsibility, must nevertheless fail because of the built-in biases of the educator and, in this case, the educating professional. Although it seems quite obvious that there is no such thing as a value-free education, and also that there is no such thing as education without its occurring in the context of life styles, social roles, personal narratives, etc., it is not an easy case to make that the attempt to foster responsibility and autonomy must of necessity fail.

The family planning nurse is caught, according to Professor Nathanson, between the dispensary functions of providing contraceptive information and methods, and the pedagogical relationship of developing a sense of personal responsibility. It is obvious to most that professionals will respond best to patients and clients who are most appropriately responsive to them, but it does not follow that there is a necessary contradiction in these two activities. Professor Nathanson says that the role of assisting women in preventing unwanted pregnancy is contradictory to the role of the family planning nurse as contributing to the development of personal moral responsibility.

If one can make the claim that autonomy is enhanced by knowledge and, of course, by increased self-knowledge, then surely this information, however transmitted, contributes in some small way to one's own personal responsibility. This might be a very small contribution, and the cultural climate in which the client operates might indeed be detrimental to the formation of that kind of responsibility. It is one thing to claim that the dispensing of contraceptive information and means gives at least a possibility of enhancing personal freedom and autonomy, but I do not believe that the claim can be made out that such dispensing is the sole or sufficient means to that autonomy. There are subcultures of all kinds in which certain sexual practices are expected and of the norm, and one's autonomy within those cultural climates is perhaps enhanced by knowing more about contraceptive means and practices, but it is difficult to claim that it is guaranteed.

If we grant to professionals, as I think we should, educational responsibilities for patients and clients, then it follows that the enormous social power of the profession needs to be examined more carefully in this context. The medicalization of contraceptive means and practices is dangerous if professionals view themselves as playing anything less than a genuine educational role. It may be the case that this process redefines inappropriate behavior from the transgression of sexual norms to the transgression of medical and bureaucratic norms, and it may also mean that because of this process professionals feel able to excuse themselves from the responsibility when those contraceptive methods fail. But I think it would be a moral mistake of the first order for any professional to absolve himself or herself from the results of his or her educational practice when that practice fails. Thus, I find it hard to see how Professor Nathanson can put together a role for family practice nurses which enables them to somehow become free of the responsibility for the careful use of the information they dispense to their patients and clients. There is a perfectly straightforward sense in which any educator has a degree, although far from complete, of responsibility for the behavior of those persons whom he or she tries to educate.

In claiming the control of adolescent pregnancy, it is the case that the medical profession risks being held accountable for behavior which it cannot fully control; but of course, in claiming responsibility for education in general, any educator risks being held accountable for behavior which he or she cannot fully control. Simply remember the charges held up against Socrates for the behavior of Alcibiades. Although no professional can be fully responsible for the behavior of his or her clients, it does not follow that there is an easy way to dodge that responsibility altogether.

I think Professor Nathanson is correct in assigning a double, dubious and highly ambiguous role to professionals, and medical professionals in particular, who try to foster personal autonomy and freedom in a relatively unbiased way, and who provide information, ideas, procedures and methods which that autonomy can use. There is always a dialectic between the attempt to create reasonably free and autonomous persons and the values imbedded in the procedures and practices which attempt to bring that freedom about. This is not an inherent contradiction; it is a problem which professionals must inevitably struggle to overcome.

Department of Philosophy
University of Missouri
Columbia, Missouri

BIBLIOGRAPHY

1. Dubler, N.: 1987, 'The Right to Fornication: The Right to Reproduce', in this volume, pp. 166–168.
2. Engelhardt, H. T., Jr.: 1987, 'Persons, Sex, and Contraception', in this volume, pp. 40–41.
3. Nathanson, C. A.: 1987, 'Family Planning and Contraceptive Responsibility', in this volume, p. 187.
4. Richards, J. R.: 1980, *The Skeptical Feminist*, Routledge and Kegan Paul, London, U.K.
5. Veatch, R. M.: 1981, *A Theory of Medical Ethics*, Basic Books, New York.

SECTION IV

CONTRACEPTION AND CHANGING IMAGES OF SEXUALITY

MEREDITH W. MICHAELS

CONTRACEPTION, FREEDOM AND DESTINY: A WOMB OF ONE'S OWN

Minor gods and goddesses also lived on Olympus besides the twelve great ones. The most powerful of them were the goddesses of destiny, Clotho, Lachesis and Atropos. They were the three Fates and they decided how long a mortal should live and how long the rule of the gods should last. When a mortal was born, Clotho spun the thread of life, Lachesis measured a certain length, and Atropos cut the thread at the end of the life. They knew the past and the future, and even Zeus had no power to sway their decisions. Their sister, Nemesis, saw to it that all evil and all good on earth were justly repaid, and all mortals feared her ([2], p. 70).

Worker . . . 3. One of the sterile females of certain social insects . . . that performs specialized work.
(*American Heritage Dictionary*)

I

"Now you can decide" says the ad, hidden in the back pages of a woman's magazine. The photograph is of a woman, taken with a pink filter to assure us that she is truly feminine, whose gaze is directed past her beringed finger into the distance. What is it that she can now decide? Not whether to have meatloaf or hotdogs, not whether to use Tide or All, not even whether to buy a house or a condominium. The ad is for contraceptive foam. The implications are enormous. Emphasize the 'now' and you become a participant in the dawn of a new age. Empha- size the "you" and you set yourself apart from those who lack this privilege and join the ranks of the liberated. Emphasize the 'can decide' and you cut the 'Fatal Thread'. It is up to you now. But what is it that has been transferred from the hands of the Fates to the hands of the woman? Look carefully when one small pressurized can is credited with lifting the veil of ignorance, the rock of Sisyphus and the burdens of destiny. Generally speaking, cans do not make people free.

The issue I wish to address is that of the relationship between contraception and reproductive freedom, particularly the sort of free- dom contraception allegedly provides women. Though it may be that women in this country are in general free from what Margaret Sanger [13] called "motherhood in bondage", it is at best naive and at worst pigheaded to assume either that it is principally to contraception that we

209

Stuart F. Spicker, William B. Bondeson, and H. Tristram Engelhardt, Jr.
The Contraceptive Ethos, 209–221.
© 1987 by D. Reidel Publishing Company.

owe thanks for this freedom or that control over reproductive sexuality is concomitant with it. Indeed, I intend to argue that women neither have, nor can experience themselves as having reproductive freedom. In order to do that I shall make the banal but often overlooked assumption that the current relationship between contraception and reproductive sexuality is rendered intelligible only if one attends to the historical and social context within which that relationship is embedded.

When one learns that in 1975 the emirs traced the drought in Northern Nigeria to the immorality of single women ([5], p. 317), it seems reasonable to speculate that the emirs' concern was not unrelated to the decline in population. The fact that single women were ordered to find husbands, and that women who were separated from their husbands were ordered to return to them, is surely more than a gratuitous act of male oppression. We have no difficulty supposing that in such a culture sexual practices, myths, beliefs and taboos are inextricably linked to other social practices and to economic needs. I do not mean to suggest that the relationship between socio-economic factors and reproductive sexuality is a straightforward one. In fact, it is clear that quite the opposite is true. Nevertheless it is easy to forget, when considering our own attitudes and practices, that they, like those of our not so distant counterparts, are in large part determined by general population needs, by infant and maternal mortality rates and by pervasive, historically rooted beliefs about the relationship between reproduction and general societal well-being. In other words, attitudes toward reproductive sexuality do not emerge by spontaneous generation, nor by forces whose operations are transparent to those upon whom they act.

Similarly, our capacity to read between the lines of other cultures, to push beyond that which appears to that which more likely is, and to understand the subtle ways in which power and control are maintained and distributed, is evident in even the most rudimentary anthropological analysis. As Garrett Hardin [4] points out, we are not lulled into believing that the Rif tribes of Northern Africa, for whom abortion is a serious offense, do not thereby practice it. Nor do we suppose that, because women in such tribes have a marketplace for abortions and contraceptives in which men are not permitted, they thereby maintain control over reproduction and hence over their status in the society. Furthermore, we chide any anthropologist who suggests that the presence of abortion and contraception, and even their appropriation by women, assures that each individual woman maintains autonomy with respect to reproductive sexuality. The stance from which we view other cultures encourages a perspective sensitive to the variety of ways in which public and private spheres are negotiated and experienced. Clearly, the standards used to determine the adequacy of an anthropologist's account of sexual practices in Vanuatu should not be abandoned when we turn to face our own.

II

In March 1983, the *New York Times* reported that the Food and Drug Administration had approved a new contraceptive device, the vaginal sponge. What the *Times* failed to report was that this device was used by the Ancient Jews in 1900 B.C., that it was endorsed by Charles Knowlton in his early nineteenth-century birth control pamphlet quaintly titled *The Fruits of Philosophy*, and that it was recommended by birth control clinics in this country in the 1930's, before the widespread availability of the diaphragm. The article in the *Times*, and countless others like it, contribute to an energetic attempt to create an aura of unprecedented creativity, progress and originality in the field of contraceptive research, an aura which is sustained by a pervasive historical and cultural myopia. It is as though contraception belonged with nuclear fission and genetic engineering on the list of nature-defying feats of contemporary science. Simultaneously, we learn that the contraceptive breakthroughs of the recent past have enabled women finally to free themselves sexually, socially and economically. Despite their apparent ideological incompatibility, both *Playboy* and *Ms. Magazine* share, in much of what they have to say on the subject, the implicit assumption that contraception itself is the remedy to a host of maladies, social and personal. Most significant is the emphasis on the idea that reproductive decisions have been transferred from Nature, the State and the Fates, to the individual woman.

The fact that contraception has been around as long as there have been people to tell about it, ought to give us pause. If we are loath to believe that women in ancient Egypt, fully equipped with spermicide-soaked sponges, had anything akin to authority in matters of reproduction, then we perhaps ought to reconsider the connection between contraception and reproductive freedom. Even a brief glance at the historical literature on birth control [3, 4, 5, 6, 8, 10] yields a list of products and procedures that is surprisingly long and marvelously inventive; that in itself is testimony to the fact that the existence of effective contraceptive measures is not dependent on the men of twentieth-century medicine. Prior to the nineteenth century, contraception was not considered to be in the province of medicine at all. One marvels at the capacity of those with only a rudimentary understanding of reproductive processes to select out of all the things there are in the world, those which are in fact effective deterrents to conception. Camel dung and vinegar do have spermicidal properties. Sponges do prevent sperm from finding their way into the uterus. Olive oil does reduce the motility of sperm. Women learned what they needed to know about contraception from their mothers, their sisters, and from the midwives who delivered their babies. It is certainly true that in the nineteenth century the picture began to change. Birth control became a matter of public concern, but in quintessential Victorian fashion, one that could not be spoken of publicly. Its public appropriation simultaneously rendered it unfit fare for private communication. It became, and largely remains, something about which even mothers and daughters cannot talk together.

It was during this time that Connecticut adopted a law prohibiting the use of contraceptives by married couples, and one senses that the law had far less to do with controlling reproductive sexual activity than it did with controlling recreational sexual activity. Though it is interesting to speculate as to how its proponents imagined the law would be enforced, one way to insure at least a modicum of compliance was to persuade people that there were no effective contraceptive methods anyway, and to make it difficult for them to discover that, in fact, there were such methods. Doctors, who were told virtually nothing about contraception in medical school, began to deliver babies, and to pleas from their patients for information, answered either "I don't know", or "I musn't tell", one of which was sure to be true. The peculiar severing of the usual lines of communication produced a combination of static and silence. If women were brave or desperate enough to talk to one another about such matters, the authority of their voices was consistently undermined by that of an emerging medical voice, one whose message was that others know better than you do about your body, but they are not always going to tell.

If this is our immediate historical legacy, then it is no wonder that we find reassuring the relative ease with which reproductive issues are discussed in the public and professional media. "If Mama won't tell me, I can find out from the *New York Times*". Nor is it surprising that we believe ourselves to have embarked on a quest of mythic proportions. We can be made to think that the contraceptive sponge is a novelty only because we have been radically severed from the past and from other cultures by a period during which ordinary sexual activity was viewed as something virtually sinful. Though we may gain comfort in thinking that we have achieved a degree of freedom in relegating such a view to the rubbish heap of history, it would perhaps behove us to attend more carefully to the conditions and the limits of that freedom. Why is it, one wonders, that the middle-class woman is permitted not only to wave her diaphragm in public but to do so under the banner of her own liberation? Similar attempts on the part of nineteenth-century feminists (who more often than not advocated not contraception but abstinence) were countered with overwhelming moral vehemence. A host of ills: promiscuity, insanity, the weakening of the democratic spirit, the abolition of motherhood and the family, and the demise of religion, were the predicted *results* of the widespread use of contraception in particular and the liberation of women in general. While there are those among us who are quite comfortable with such predictions, the rest of us view them as figments of the overzealous Victorian imagination. Women have requested, demanded, and pleaded for control, or something close to it, over reproductive sexuality. Is it that their right to such control has finally been established, that the clear light of reason has finally broken through the darkness of history?

In order to temper the spirit with which we answer such a question, we need only recall the Rif tribes. Surely, there we feel obliged to consider the larger context in which reproductive policies are adjudicated and maintained. If reproduction in this country is, in general, no longer seen as the inevitable fate of women, it is in large part because women have been called to other tasks. The level of individual prosperity that the middle class has come to expect is no longer attainable without the economic contributions of women. Our expectations, for ourselves and our children, cannot be met with one income alone. The houses in which we live, the sneakers on our feet, the television sets in our living rooms, the bicycles in our garages, and the colleges our children attend are increasingly purchased by money brought into the family by the working mother. If economic prosperity is held as an absolute value, then, when it is threatened, we will make those accommodations requisite to its preservation. Since it currently cannot be maintained if women at home are producing further drains on the economic system, they will not only be permitted, but encouraged to enter the marketplace and to control the rate at which they produce children. When a host organism begins to discover that what was a beneficial symbiosis has instead become antagonistic, it is quite likely to alter the terms of the relationship with its parasites. This is particularly true in cases, where the parasites that once served to sustain the host, now begin to drain its life blood.

To suppose that the availability of contraception itself places reproductive decisions in the hands of individual women is to suppose that individual liberty can emerge independently of social and economic constraints. While it is true that women are free from the burdens of unrestricted reproduction, that freedom is not based on the conferral of a right to reproductive control. For that reason, it is a tenuous freedom, one which can be revoked if it is no longer in the interests of those in whose province the assignment of benefits and burdens lies. Rights and liberties come and go, reproduction is always with us. Of course, when one views the matter from the perspective of society as a whole, it should come as no surprise that a phenomenon as central as reproduction is tied to forces well beyond the control of individuals, particularly individuals to whom control of any kind has never been fully granted. The reproductive freedom currently enjoyed by women is thus conditional, both in its nature and in its extent. If we have trouble recognizing this, it is because the conditions under which it has been granted are obscured by a willful historical inattention. Women have long asked for more extensive control over reproduction. The fact that it has recently been given them does not entail that their right to it has finally been recognized.

III

If reproductive freedom occupies an ambiguous position in moral space, then it should come as no surprise that women fail to see as straightforward the choice of whether or not to reproduce. In 1920, Margaret Sanger claimed that "No woman can call herself free until she can consciously choose whether she will or will not be a mother" ([12], p. 94). In 1929, Virginia Woolf claimed that no woman can call herself free unless she has five hundred a year and a room of her own [14]. Sanger and Woolf, though their emphases differ, are nevertheless concerned to establish what they take to be the conditions that would enable women to abandon their posts at the margins of society. Each stands at the outside looking in and each, it appears, has something of a remedy: for Woolf, it is a room of one's own; for Sanger, it is a womb of one's own. It is by examining the intersection of these apparently disparate remedies that we can perhaps come to understand the impediments to freedom. To put it somewhat cryptically, in order for the reproductive choice to be one that is indeed consciously made (as Sanger insists it must be), a woman must have, must really have, a room of her own. On the other hand, in order for a woman to have a room of her own, the reproductive choice must be one she makes consciously.

When the ad for contraceptive foam urges us to believe that The Decision is now in our hands, why is it that the claim does not ring true? I have already attempted to explain the ways in which reproductive decisions fail to be ones over which individuals have control. Nevertheless, that explanation is fully compatible with the view that, in spite of the forces that shape and maintain assignments of control in the reproductive sphere, women can experience themselves as exercising control over a matter that is, in some sense, strictly private. What I now wish to show is why they do not in general do so. I have in mind as a paradigm case the woman who is well-established in a career, who has no children and who now, at the age of thirty or so, decides that the time for decision is upon her. That there are infinite variations on this paradigm will not, I hope, detract from the point I wish to make. In order to dispel confusion, I want to make it clear that I in no way wish to underestimate the crucial role played by contraception in establishing reproductive choice. Without ready access to it, it would not be possible to postpone indefinitely the decision whether to be a mother. The woman whose ambitions carry her into the highly competitive world of commerce cannot hope to succeed unless her energies are focused on little else. It is surely true that contraception enables women to choose and then to negotiate that path with the singlemindedness it demands. What is less clear is that the freedom to make such a choice is tantamount to *reproductive* freedom.

In order to make that point, I will enlist the services of Alasdair MacIntyre. In *After Virtue* [7], MacIntyre presents a conceptual scheme whose purpose it is to elucidate the nature of human action and, with it, personal identity. MacIntyre's claim is that in order properly to understand either, we must see individual actions in the context of the unity of an individual life. The unity of an individual life can itself be understood only in the context of what he calls "settings", namely, human institutions and practices. But what ties all of this machinery together, according to MacIntyre, is the fact that any human action is an enacted narrative.

. . . in successfully identifying and understanding what someone else is doing we always move toward placing a particular episode in the context of a set of narrative histories, histories both of the individuals concerned and of the settings in which they act and suffer ([7], p. 197).

To the question, "What are you doing?" I might answer, "Playing with my computer", "Trying to figure out the best way to put my point", "Writing a paper", "Trying to get tenure", "Working to feed my family", or "Avoiding the phone call to my mother". Each one of those responses renders my action intelligible by setting it in a context, a context that is properly described by a narrative history. In each case, the action being performed is situated in an individual life which is itself situated in a narrative history that transcends the boundaries of that life. If my intention is best described as that of attempting to get tenure, the intention itself can be understood only with reference to a practice in which colleges and universities engage, a practice which can only be understood with reference to the goals of such institutions. By the time we have reached the circumference of embeddings, we are well beyond the action with which we began. And yet, it should be clear that the action is intelligible only within their sphere.

If narrative supplies the link between individual actions and individual lives, and between individual lives and human institutions, then stories are not only told, but also lived.

I can only answer the question 'What am I to do?' if I can answer the prior question 'Of what story or stories do I find myself a part?' We enter human society, that is, with one or more imputed characters – roles into which we have been drafted – and we have to learn what they are in order to be able to understand how others respond to us and how our responses to them are apt to be construed. It is through hearing stories. . . that children learn or mislearn what a child and what a parent is, what the cast of characters may be in the drama into which they have been born and what the ways of the world are" ([7], p. 201).

The stories we are told, the characters whose narratives we enter in virtue of being born when and where we are, will inevitably determine the narratives by means of which we can render intelligible our own intentions, actions and choices. Certain narratives are not open to me: I cannot choose to be a Soviet Georgian, living on yogurt and clean air; I cannot choose to be a famous coloratura; I cannot choose to be a linebacker for the Minnesota Vikings. I cannot even choose to be a flight attendant. Though the sense in which I intend this will, I trust, become somewhat more clear as I go on, I want to emphasize that the fact that I cannot choose to be a flight attendant is not due to ungenerosity on the part of the airlines. Nor do I mean to suggest that there are no circumstances under which I might find that alternative the best, or the only one available to me. What I do mean is that the narratives I am currently enacting do not include me as a character, now willingly and consciously choosing to be a flight attendant. This is due in part to features of me and in part to features of my circumstances.

It is here that we return to the story of the woman who has chosen as her primary role that of the successful participant in the marketplace. Down to its smallest detail, the narrative she enacts is one whose history does not include women, though it works hard to accommodate recognized differences in the concerns and needs of males and females. Bill Blass designs suits for men and women, Ferragamo makes shoes for the female executive, O.B. makes tampons that can be transferred discretely from briefcase to closed palm. Each one of these provides women with a sense that the story into which she has entered can bend itself in her direction. But it is important to note that this is indeed a narrative she has chosen to enter, not one into which she was born, not one she inherited in virtue of being a woman.

In anyone's life there are moments at which he feels he has forgotten his lines, that the curtain has risen on a stammering and fretful actor. For a woman who spends much of her day in a world that was neither designed by her, nor with her in mind, it is not that she forgets her lines, for she was never told what her lines would be. She dresses up in her father's clothes and goes to work, a place that appears as alien to her as an adult participant as it did to her as a childhood observer. She has been invited to tea and might at any moment be caught with egg on her face and be asked to leave.

Now surely there is a sense in which the experiences of the woman here described are like those of anyone who steps into an ongoing narrative, whose participants do not expect to find him there. And, indeed, the difficulties are likely to proliferate when the person has chosen to step in and has not, as it were, been left on the doorstep. Yet when the person is a member of a group which has systematically been denied access to unconstrained participation in an activity central to the culture in which she lives, her decision to participate is one she must make over and over again. The narrative into which she is born pre-dominates, and it is only by a continual act of will that she has tran-scended its boundaries. I have in mind, of course, the narrative history of motherhood. The woman who chooses to enact an unfamiliar narra-tive and thereby chooses not to bow to necessity feels herself standing alone, an individual without a history and with an uncertain future. Hannah Arendt puts it this way:

Nothing indeed can be more frightening than the notion of solipsistic freedom – the 'feeling' that my standing apart, isolated from everyone else, is due to free will, that nothing and nobody can be held responsible for it but me myself . . . . Isn't trust in necessity, the conviction that everything is as 'it was to be' infinitely preferable to freedom bought at the price of contingency?" ([1], pp. 195–196)

Though the narrative history of motherhood encloses all of us, women exist at its center, and men, in virtue of the fact that they are nurtured by, but cannot be, mothers, exist at its margins. It is by reference to that narrative that so many actions of women are rendered intelligible, both to themselves and to others. Every time a woman takes her pill, puts in her diaphragm, uses her foam, she does so in order to fend off the pull of destiny. Her effort to join with men at the margins of the enclosing narrative is one which requires the uninterrupted vigilence of her will. There is always the fear, not that her diaphragm will leak, but that her will, whose ancestors were weakened from want of exercise, might crumble under the strain. The defiance in the voice of young women who construe themselves not merely to be choosing careers but to be rejecting motherhood is surely a product of their effort to escape the boundaries of a narrative to which they are unwilling heirs.

IV

The sometimes nagging, sometimes beseeching, sometimes seductive voice with which motherhood tells its story is impossible to quiet. It appears always as the voice of destiny, accompanied by a Nemesis who promises retribution for wrongs committed. Polymorphous and adap-tive, this Nemesis can appear in a variety of guises. For Elizabeth Stuart Phelps (1815–1852), the struggle to balance motherhood with a writing career was experienced as the struggle between good and evil:

There are *two* angels . . . the angel over the right shoulder who records for God every evidence of right mothering, of 'performing faithfully all those little household cares and duties on which the comfort and the virtue of her family depend'; and the awful angel over the left shoulder who, weeping, records for God every bit of time not so used, every lapse and deficiency ([9], p. 207).

For Adrienne Rich (c. 1965), who was engaged in a similar struggle, the Nemesis appears not as an agent of God sitting outside her, but in good post-Freudian fashion as a part of her very self: "Sometimes I seem to myself, in my feelings toward these tiny guiltless beings, a monster of selfishness and intolerance," and "Perhaps one is a monster – an anti-woman – something driven and without recourse to the normal and appealing consolations of love, motherhood and joy in others" ([11], pp. 1–2). The woman who stands at the edge of the narrative history of motherhood, trying to decide whether to step in, knows that she has already failed, that she long ago opened the door to monsters and avenging angels. If she chooses motherhood, she will fail to be a true mother; if she chooses otherwise, she fails to be a true woman. Indeed, it is part of the age-old story of motherhood that one does not choose to enter it by conscious decision but rather by allowing nature to run its course. Thus, the mere fact of making a decision is the woman's first indication that she cannot make the right one. It is here that my inability to choose to be a flight attendant is perhaps cast in a clearer light. Given the narrative history of flight attendants, that they are woman who can smile under duress, who do not mind flying, who enjoy spending short periods of time in many different places, who can tolerate being fondled by strange men, who perhaps fantasize about marrying pilots and so on, I cannot choose to be such a person, for that is not the sort of person I am. I could play the role, pretending that such things are true of me. But I would know all along that they are not, that it is all, in some sense, a ruse. I am the one who is cheating because I am the one who is enacting a role that I know I cannot truly be. And so it is with the woman. The sort of person she has become is the sort of person who cannot do more than pretend to be a mother.

The sort of impossibility here referred to is obviously not logical, nor even psychological, impossibility. It is rather narrative impossibility. The alternative roles women choose to occupy do not fit comfortably within the boundaries of the narrative history of motherhood, a narrative they bring with them simply in virtue of being women. It is no wonder, then, that a woman who has, for years, successfully transcended those boundaries will find herself in never-never land when she finally decides to consider whether she is now ready to be a mother. For the decision to become a mother is one which does not simply require the construction of a narrative which coexists peaceably with the one in which she currently finds herself. The stories she has been told and the ones she has lived make it clear that motherhood is not a hobby designed for weekend amusement. Its narrative is rich, full and apparently all-encompassing. To enter it is to become a different person, indeed, the person who, by an effort of will, she deliberately left behind. It is a narrative that does not include within it as protaganists women who occupy other, equally demanding roles. If one chooses to enter it, hoping to take along all that one is, one must do so blind and unscripted. When a woman turns on the radio and hears T. Berry Brazelton, his voice resonant with authority, telling her that mother-child bonding is guaranteed only if the mother is fully available to the child for a year, that sometimes it occurs in only six months (but you never can tell), she is once again confronted with the fact that the life she has been living up until now cannot include her as the mother she ought to be. Mothers are people who think first of their children, are there uninterruptedly for the first year, wait every afternoon for the school bus, have infinite patience with lost socks and spilled juice, and understand that they are simply and absolutely subordinate in importance to their children. Because the properties essential to the story of motherhood are not ones she can hope to have, the woman bears to mothers the relation that I bear to flight attendants. She can pretend to be a mother, but she cannot really be one. But for her the stakes are higher, both because they involve not merely the momentary comfort of airline passengers, but the continuous psychological well-being of her child, and because motherhood inevitably surfaces at the center of a woman's identity, while flight-attendanthood does not.

Freedom within this context is of course never absolute. We are constrained by the narratives we inherit, the ones in which we find ourselves by reason of accident or misjudgment, and even by the boundaries of those we willingly inhabit. There is no such thing as sole authorship, for no one stands outside of history and of culture. Freedom resides rather in the capacity to participate fully and consciously in the creation of variations and nuances, subplots and sidetracks on and in the narratives that constitute one's historical legacy. To find oneself more controlled by than controlling the terms under which one enters into and then participates in that legacy, is to find oneself radically and painfully unfree. Contraception alone does not provide the conditions requisite for freedom. If it assures women that the reproductive decisions they make can in fact be carried out, it does nothing to assure them that the decisions themselves are within their control.

To shut the door on the voices of destiny, one needs a room of one's own. Woolf's room was one in which Shakespeare's sister could finally write her poems. The room I have in mind is the one in which each woman can write a narrative whose principal character chooses consciously, and hence freely, whether to be a mother or not. Only when she can do that will there be a clear path between contraception and reproductive freedom.

Hampshire College
Amherst, Massachusetts

BIBLIOGRAPHY

1. Arendt, H.: 1981, *The Life of the Mind*, Harcourt Brace Jovanovich, New York, N.Y.
2. D'Aulaire, I. and D'Aulaire, E.: 1962, *Book of Greek Myths*, Doubleday, New York, N.Y.
3. Gordon, L.: 1977, *Woman's Body, Woman's Right*, Penguin, New York, N.Y.
4. Hanssen-Jurreit, M.: 1982, *Sexism: The Male Monopoly on History and Thought*, Farrar, Straus and Giroux, New York, N.Y.
5. Hardin, G. (ed.): 1969, *Population, Birth Control and Evolution*, W. H. Freeman, San Francisco, Calif.
6. Knowlton, C.: 1838, 'The Fruits of Philosophy,' in Rothman, D. J. and S. M. (eds.), 1972, *Birth Control Morality in Nineteenth Century America*, Arno Press, New York, N.Y. ·
7. MacIntyre, A.: 1981, *After Virtue*, Notre Dame University Press, Notre Dame, Ind.
8. McLaren, A.: 1978, *Birth Control in Nineteenth-Century England*, Holmes and Meier, New York, N.Y.
9. Olsen, T.: 1979, *Silences*, Delta, Seymour Lawrence, New York, N.Y.
10. Reed, J.: 1978, *From Private Vice to Public Virtue*, Basic Books, New York, N.Y.
11. Rich, A.: 1977, *Of Woman Born*, Bantam, New York, N.Y.
12. Sanger, M.: 1920, *Woman and the New Race*, Brentano, New York, N.Y.
13. Sanger, M.: 1928, *Motherhood in Bondage,* Brentano, New York, N.Y.
14. Woolf, V.: 1929, *A Room of One's Own*, Harcourt Brace Jovanovich, New York, N.Y.

ROBERT C. SOLOMON

SEX, CONTRACEPTION AND CONCEPTIONS OF SEX

> . . . males and females united without any premeditated design, as chance, occasion, or desire brought them together, nor had they any great occasion for language to make known what they had to say to each other. They parted with the same ease.
>
> Jean-Jacques Rousseau, [16]

There is the myth: 'free sex', as told by a philosophical libertine who practiced it freely. It is a distinctively male fantasy, of course; one might say, a paradigm of irresponsibility. But suppose the problem of unwanted pregnancy – and to see as a problem at all is already an enormous philosophical and political leap – could be solved. Could sex not then become as Jean-Jacques fantasized it, 'free' and divorced from morals and even manners? "Liberated from our biology" as Shulamith Firestone once put it: how different would our sexual world be?[5].

Does effective contraceptive technology alter our conception of sex? Does it 'free' sex from extraneous fears and moral concerns? When I started my research into the topic, I thought I knew; what had had a more direct and dramatic effect on sexual conduct than the availability of the pill in the 1960s, and what could be more obvious than the 'sexual revolution' then set in motion? But on further investigation and reflection, I began to realize that our modern medical miracles had ancient, however less effective counterparts, and that sexual revolutions, looking at the whole of history, have been a dime-a-dozen. With that in mind, and without lacking gratitude for the advances of modern medicine, I want to answer the question with a qualified 'No.' Our new contraceptive technology has not altered our conceptions of sex in anything like the radical 'revolutionary' ways we sometimes imagine.

> Sexual intercourse began
> In nineteen sixty-three
> (Which was rather late for me) –
> Between the end of the CHATTERLEY ban
> And the Beatles' first LP.
>
> Philip Larkin,
> HIGH WINDOWS [10]

223

Stuart F. Spicker, William B. Bondeson, and H. Tristram Engelhardt, Jr.
The Contraceptive Ethos, 223–240.
© 1987 *by D. Reidel Publishing Company.*

I would like to throw open to question the concept taken most for granted in contemporary discussions of contraception – sex. For a philosopher to even ask 'what, really, is sex?' is to open him or herself up to ridicule. (Who else would ask such a question?) 'What is the problem?' it is replied curtly, with a smirk, occasionally coupled with an offer of an ostensive definition. "Sex is, – well, sex is – just what it is". It is straightforward biology, which happens (usually) to involve two people, and, more importantly, which happens to be fun. Unfortunately, fun has its price, for nature's purpose is not the same as our purposes. But, fortunately, in sex as in so much of modern life, human technology has taken control of nature. Sex is one thing; reproduction is something else. A thousand generations have enjoyed one only along with the other. We, finally, have separated them.

Reproduction, because it involves the lives of other human beings in the most dramatic way imaginable, their very creation, is at the center of our moral concerns; indeed, until recently, the very concept of a person's 'morals' was far more concerned with his or her sexual behavior than with any other virtues or vices. But now, severing sex and reproduction, also threatens to divorce sex and morals, according to the fears of many contemporary moralists. In fact, this has not happened. What current technology, coupled with the current sexual counter revolution, shows us is that sexuality is still at the heart of morality, and though there are the most serious questions of life and death involved in questions of reproduction there remain equally ethical – if not so mortal – questions of morals in our non-reproductive conception of sex. Sex, in other words, is not as 'free' as the sexual revolutionaries once thought.

What is sex? It is, in some sense, the coupling of bodies in certain, not so strictly circumscribed ways. There is a central paradigm, which provides the continuity with most of the animal kingdom and even a small minority of plants – heterosexual intercourse. Indeed, given the flat and untitillating use of the word 'sex' in biology textbooks to describe the behavior of scorpions and fish, not to mention pine trees, one gets the idea that sex for us is much the same physical process, except that we alone in the kingdoms of life have chosen to make a moral issue of it. But this is wholly misleading, if it is not actually fraudulent. In fact, most human sex has about as much continuity with arachnids and dicotyledons as eating the Sunday wafer and sipping the Passover wine have to do with nutrition.

Sex is ideas. Sex is not about conception – at least, not usually; our conceptions about sex are far more tied to our morals than our gonads, though, to be sure, one can easily and amusingly imagine how different our sexual fantasies might be if our organs were differently constituted, say, on the bottom of one foot or – reminiscent of a once popular but physiologically dubious movie – inside of the mouth or the throat. This essay, accordingly, is about our sexual conceptions, not about conception or contraception as such. Indeed, what continues to strike me as remarkable is that, despite the dramatic developments two decades ago, changes in contraceptive technology are not the major determinants of our conceptions of sex. My historical thesis in a nutshell: attitudes about sex determine the acceptability of contraception, at least as much as the availability of effective contraception determines attitudes about sex.

1. THE TELEOLOGY OF SEX; THE PURPOSE OF SEX

Sex is not just 'matter in motion' (we may refrain from mentioning the many more imaginative metaphors), plus the pleasurable sensations thereby promoted and produced. Sex, like virtually all human activities and like most biological phenomena, has a purpose, or purposes. In the perspective of biology, of course, that purpose is clear enough: the perpetuation of the species. Pleasure, the expression or the stimulation of romantic love, getting even with the husband or getting a good grade the hard way are at most epiphenomena, perhaps effective motivation, but probably of no real relevance at all. Yet only rarely, if ever, does one 'have sex' within the biological perspective. The purpose of sex is therefore only rarely, if ever, the same as 'nature's purpose' – the perpetuation of the species. There is also OUR purpose or purposes, what we desire over and above – or instead of – fulfilling our biological roles as self-perpetuating links in a chain that extends from Adam and Eve or perhaps rather Lucy to Nietzsche's *übermensch* or 'the last man.'

Philosophers – following the ancient Greeks – like to refer to the purpose of a phenomenon as its 'telos'; thus we can speak of the 'teleology of sex' – its ultimate purpose. But our teleology immediately splits at least in two, for there is what we have called, with evolutionary naivete, 'nature's purpose,' and then there are our various purposes, which are not the same thing. Indeed, once we introduce that distinction, we immediately begin to wonder how the two have ever been connected, except for the contingencies of biology – in the same way that one might wonder how it is that the miracle that we call 'language' has such an intimate connection with the organ of ingestion (Jacques Derrida aside, I should add).

a. 'Nature's Purpose'

To talk of 'nature's purpose' is, of course, naive. We no longer talk so easily of the teleology of the world – as Aristotle did so long ago [1] and as Hegel and his henchmen did with less ease a century and a half ago. We prefer causal models, efficient rather than final causes, physio-chemical processes rather than instincts and collectively unconscious cunning. Nevertheless, we can say, uncontroversially but a bit oddly, that sex does serve a purpose – whether or not we want to say that sex has a purpose. Sex provides – for the moment – the only means of reproduction of human beings, though whether this is a good thing in the eyes of some larger telos is an awesome question I would not want to broach here. And sometimes, about 2.3 periods per lifetime for most Americans, considerably less for many couples in other cultures whose birth rate is inversely higher, nature's purpose does indeed coincide with at least one of the purposes of the heterosexual couple having intercourse. (It is logically possible, of course, that a homosexual couple might also adopt this telos, but this possibility is not a fruitful topic of discussion.) This happy harmony is not our concern here, however; it is the divorce rather than the marriage of sex and conception that interests us. Let us turn, therefore, to persons' purposes, leaving nature to fend for herself.

b. Persons' Purposes

It is with persons' purposes that the teleology of sex becomes complicated. I have not mentioned some parallel complications in nature, for example, male dogs or chimps mounting other males, not in procreative confusion but as an unchallengable gesture of dominance. I do want to consider such behavior, however, in the context of human sexuality. To take a more common example, it is often said, in many languages, that to have intercourse with a woman is to 'possess' her. I do not take such talk lightly, and the fact that the woman in question may or may not conceive as the result of the possessive act does not seem to be relevant to the matter. I choose this somewhat feudal example to underscore the sometimes less-than-romantic theme of the theory that I will be presenting here; sex is not, in addition to its biological functions, just a matter of pleasure or the expression of love. The human purposes of sex are spread across an enormous range of symbolic and practical concerns, from love and intentional debasement to a mere sleep aid. To talk about 'the purpose' of sex, even confining ourselves to 'our purposes' is a serious mistake. It does not follow, however, that this diversity makes impossible a unified theory of sexuality. Indeed, it is the diversity itself that has to be explained.

By 'persons' purposes,' I do not mean conscious purposes, nor, of course, do I refer only to explicit and mutually agreed upon purposes. The cooperative telos of the transparently self-reflective and psychologically explicit sado-masochist couple is one thing; the fumbling, confused clash of desires, fantasies, habits, expectations and aims that most of us take to bed with us is quite different as well as more common. Indeed, it is part of the ethics of sex (as opposed to the ethics of reproduction) that most of our purposes remain unspoken; it is a matter of curiosity as well as 'liberation' that we have recently been encouraged to make explicit our fantasies and desires. Not surprisingly, most of these tend to be rather mechanical ('touch me here') rather than the more significant messages and meanings that such behavior expresses, knowingly or not.

I do not want to attack the profound question of 'the unconscious,' much less the even more problematic Jungian notion of a 'collective' unconscious. There is no doubt that such a thing, consisting at least of those most basic biological impulses and residual instincts, which Kraft-Ebbing misleadingly calls 'the 6th, genital sense.' But whether there is an extinct-laden unconscious is quite another matter, and at least one proto-Jungian philosopher, Nietzsche, [12] vehemently denied the collectivity of our impulses, turning the tables to insist that our 'herd-consciousness' is to be found in consciousness, our individuality in our instincts [13]. Our own view of sexuality, as opposed to some of our theories about it, seems to side with Nietzsche. Each of us appears to belabor the illusion – against all evidence – that each of us is sexually unique. But – back to the point – many of our purposes, individual or collective, instinctual or learned, are not conscious. When told about them – if we have not already been too jaded by 80 years of Freud – we would probably deny them, or, at least, dismiss them as minor aberrations, and 'out of character.'

2. WHAT DO I WANT WHEN I WANT YOU?

Any discussion of human sexuality involves more than a catalog of organs, feelings, physiological and behavioral responses; sex is first of all desire, both temporally and, less obviously, phenomenologically. Indeed, one might make a case that sex without desire is not sexuality at all, though one hesitates to suggest or imagine what it might be. But what is it that one desires?

The glib answers are soon forthcoming, along with that familiar smirk and a number of rude responses. Such responses, however, are largely limited to adolescents and academic seminars. A novice may think that the 'end' (telos as well as terminus) of sex is successful intercourse (though even the notion of 'success' should be carefully scrutinized here). But clearly despite certain philosophical protests, sex is not one of those activities that is 'desired for its own sake' (if anything is so desired). It is not just that sex sometimes serves a telos, but that it always does. If there is anything like a purely sexual impulse (and they are very rare if they exist in us at all), we still have to say something such as 'it is the satisfaction of the impulse' that is in question, not sex for sex's sake. Indeed, we should want to know more about this alleged 'impulse' (which was 'discovered' or 'postulated', in fact fabricated – at the end of the 19th century). Some animals perhaps may experience something like 'pure sexual desire,' but this is noteworthy only insofar as it is also isolated and empty, virtually unrelated to any other activities and something of a mystery to the animal itself. Dennett, in an unusual bit of anthropomorphizing, imagines a bird in the midst of its instinctual behavior, musing to itself, 'Why am I doing this?' Clearly few mammals enjoy such an impulse; sex becomes a matter of status as well as species-preservation, and, watching my male dog's behavior around a female in heat, it is clear that sexual desire supplies only a small if not minimal motive, and is interwoven inseparably with a half dozen other concerns. When we return to human sexuality, we might be far closer to the mark by beginning, not with the obvious but with the obscure, not with the simple-minded aim of wanting intercourse but with the 'infinite yearning' of eros suggested by Aristophanes in Plato's Symposium [14]. In philosophy, it is always better to err towards the infinite than to get trapped in the picayune.

So, what is sexual desire? Indeed, is it possible (as Michel Foucault hints [6]) that we ought to give up such talk as quite misleading and mythological, as if sex were indeed a distinct and isolated impulse with only the most peculiar and often antagonistic connections with our other motives and desires? Without going quite so far, we can begin to appreciate the complexity of what we call 'sexual desire' and its intricate connections with other desires and motives. Sex is not a distinct activity, except according to certain customs and rituals which make it so. Accordingly, sexual desire is not an easily distinguished mode of desire – which is how it is possible to produce those yearly disclosures that football, Pac-Man, quoits, metaphysics, process philosophy and eating artichokes are sexual. Who can say where one desire starts and another ends? How is it that Eric Rohmer's obsessive desire to touch Claire's Knee is highly sexual while the practiced intercourse of a jaded Don Juan may be just about as sexual as his desire to get it over with and go home to watch the Tonight Show? When we begin to analyse sexual desire, therefore, we should not be surprised that there is much more to it than sex. Indeed, sometimes sex might not even be part of it at all.

How could this be? And what does it have to do with the topic of contraception and conceptions of sex. First of all, the example of Claire's Knee – and if that sounds too fantastic consider your day-to-day furtive glance around the office – shows, if not yet convincingly, that the end of sex and sexual desire need not be sexual intercourse. Indeed, one might be obsessed with sex but find the very idea of intercourse unthinkable. One should therefore not leap to the now nearly automatic conclusion that such a desire must be 'repressed' or 'suppressed' or any other 'pressed' including 'un-ex-pressed.' If sexual desire is not necessarily aimed at intercourse – heterosexual intercourse in particular – then the supposed essential tie between sex and sexual desire and those rather constricted activities in which pregnancy is possible is dramatically weakened. This is not to deny that most heterosexual couplings do end (terminus if not telos) in intercourse of the most often-prescribed variety. It is only to say that sexual desire is not so firmly connected to intercourse as is often supposed. Our sexual conceptions are far more independent of considerations concerning the consequences of intercourse than the linkage between contraceptive technology and sexual freedom suggests.

3. FUNCTIONALISM

In a society schooled in efficiency, in which ethics and utility are often thought to be the same, in which even physical exercise is supposed to serve a purpose, we should not be surprised that our conceptions of sex tend to turn to questions of function – to the uses of sex. My discussion of the teleology of sex might be viewed as part and parcel of this pragmatist orientation, and desirable as it might seem 'for its own sake,' sex in America is almost always defended in terms of some further goal – good health, happiness and interpersonal satisfaction. The idea of chastity horrifies us, and medical science has not been slow to catalog through the ages the various malfunctions that cruelly follow this unnatural abstinence.

Yet, the pragmatic notion of 'having a function', like the more classical notion of teleology, is not a singular notion. It admits a variety of interpretations, from the traditional biological accounts of 'instinct' and 'species preservation' (that is, 'nature's purpose' – serving that natural function), to the Freudian account of pleasure as the purpose, however construed, in terms of the hydraulics of the 'psychic apparatus,' not the phenomenal sensations of 'fun.' But of particular interest to us here is the first of these interpretations, sex's natural function, reproduction. (Note that "procreation," even in the word itself, takes us at least one infinite step beyond nature.) What are we to make of the inescapably close connection – some philosophers even suggest entailment – between sexual desire and heterosexual intercourse?

The standard view, I take it, is this: sexuality changes with changes in its circumstances, the technology of contraception in particular. Taken as a hypothesis, the view suggests the following reading of history: in epochs where contraception is effective and available, sex is plentiful, relatively unrepressed and 'free.' Where contraception is not effective or available, sex tends to be prohibited, timid and fearful. But even a casual reading of the literature shows that not only is this hypothesis wrong, but its very foundation is upsidedown. (I refer here to the study by John Reed[s] who demonstrates this hypothesis with intriguing detail). The correlation between contraceptive efficiency and sexual attitudes is most unclear; indeed there are cultures with no 'protection' against pregnancy that are highly promiscuous, and just as many cultures with relatively effective contraception that are, in our terms, 'Victorian.' (Oddly enough, many of the actual Victorians fall into the first class, rather than the second.) Thus the whole notion that contraceptive apparatus determines the nature of sexuality is inverted; it is rather attitudes towards sexuality – and, of course, attitudes towards population growth and the practicalities of having children – that determine the interest in, the effectiveness of, and the availability of contraception. Of course, there are societies in which readily available contraception is withheld from the public precisely in order to counteract a casual or promiscuous attitude towards sexuality. Witness the Reagan Administration's abortive and stupidly misconceived 'Squeal Rule', according to which the parents of a young girl must be notified if she is to receive birth control information. Conservatives quickly respond, though for the wrong reasons, that information about birth control has not proven to lower the bastard birth rate, and some come to the correct conclusion – though with the wrong motives – that attitudes toward sex are not determined and are not therefore alterable through technological know-how alone. But these are standard twists and turns in the history of sexuality, not its primary path. It is the utter failure of the 'Squeal Rule,' not its paternalistic intentions, that has made us aware that sexual attitudes do not depend on technological availability; technological availability pivots on sexual attitudes, in this case, an atavistic nostalgia for the days of virginity, when sex was more feared than desired.

Functionalism, crudely conceived, is the view that sex serves the conveniences of life; it is desired when it is convenient, not desired when inconvenient, with contraception high on the list of conveniences. This is, however, a crude view of sex, and a crude view of life as well. Again let's remember Aristophanes' reference to eros as an 'infinite yearning,' [14]. We will not understand that yearning unless we give up the functional, as well as the biological, view of sex.

4. WHAT IS 'SEX'?

The genealogy of 'sex' begins, no doubt, with the birds and the bees. But it is a thin 'natural' history of love that does not soon see that the very word 'natural' – in a cultural context – is a *moral* term. 'Nature' might aim at propagation of the genotype, but cultures are concerned with group solidarity, rank and status, rules, respect and, for the sake of authority as well as order, prohibitions. To think that all of this is functional in the crude sense, aimed at population control or convenience, is nonsense. Indeed, much of the history of the availability of contraception is the history of power politics: the priests against the witches, the Republicans against the remnants of the counter-culture. What is 'natural' depends not on biology but on ideology.

Our concept of 'nature' is inherited from Aristotle, the Greeks, the church, the Enlightenment. In all of its forms, it displays one of the more glamorous sophistries in Western thinking: the appeal to a silent and therefore incontrovertible Nature in the defense of particularly provincial practices. Indeed, it is rarely biological nature that is in question; it is more usually 'natural reason', which is, as often suggested, most unnatural, even 'a bit of the divine'. When philosophers sought a 'natural religion', 'for example, they were not after nature worship or what Santayana called 'animal faith'; they were after rational arguments. And when there are demands for 'natural sex', it is not bestiality or rear-entry intercourse that is preferred; the call is rather to 'rational sex', which means, that for which there are accepted standards and arguments (most notably what I have elsewhere called "the two-minute emissionary-missionary male-superior ejaculation service", with some credit to John Barth). Whether or not sex is the danger to civilization that Freud thought it was, the traditional emphasis has been on quick and efficient sex, just enough to satisfy what D. H. Lawrence called 'evacuation lust' and, in the larger scheme of things, to ensure an adequate supply of progeny to maintain the status quo. Indeed, in our genealogy of sex and 'sex', we should look to the social politics of classes and inheritance rights before the technological availability of contraception.

What then is sex? Like most loaded terms in our vocabulary, 'sex' defies definition. It is rather a political term, to be used in ways more defined by power than by established semantics. Like most loaded philosophical terms, it shifts, suspiciously, between an indisputable paradigm and abstract arguments of the sort we have gotten used to since Kraft-Ebbing and Freud. The paradigm is heterosexual· intercourse, embellished with perhaps minimal preparatory passion ('foreplay') and typically succeeded by sleep or television rather than pregnancy. One might say, following some Oxford philosophers, that 'if that isn't sex, nothing is'. Perhaps, but the difficult task, hidden in this paradigm case argument, is to specify the feature of that paradigm. Is it the presence of male and female, or just the presence of two people? Is orgasm necessary to the paradigm? For both or only for the male? Is ejaculation of the male sufficient? (Ejaculation being the physical event of which orgasm is the more holistic phenomenon). Must two people go 'all the way' or is it sufficient just that they want to? Indeed, is it even necessary for the paradigm that the genitals are the focus of attention, though, as a matter of contingency, we might quickly note that there are certain non-logical advantages to their inclusion.

'Sex' is a plastic, political term; the presence of an indisputable paradigm does not lessen its flexibility or its controversiality. The test case, perhaps, will always be homosexuality. Is it included in the paradigm? Does it count in a culture as 'natural sex'? In our own society, there are clearly no agreed upon answers to these questions. But before we try to tighten the link between ideological questions about sexual conceptions and technological questions about contraception, we should focus our attention on homosexuality. Here is, to say the obvious, a mode of sexuality in which pregnancy and contraception are not issues. But what we find is that homosexuality displays a history that is parallel to and usually a part of the history of heterosexuality. Its values are typically the same. Even its gestures and gender (not sex) identities are the same. To say that this is because it models itself after heterosexuality is to betray both a bias and a woeful historical blindness. Indeed, the most celebrated example of a homosexual culture – the ancient Greeks – despised women and heterosexuality, so much so that, in Plato's symposium [14] virtually all of the speakers take pains to point out the inferiority of that merely functional domestic *eros* in contrast to the divine status of that 'higher' *eros* between men (more properly, between youths and men). What do we find when we look at Greek homosexuality – a licentious free-for-all with no restrictions, given the irrelevance of conception? Not at all. Indeed, the best books on the subject [4] as well as the ancient texts themselves show us quite clearly that the sexual ethic among the Greeks was, if anything, more precise and much less hypocritical than the sexual mores of modern heterosexual cultures. Again, sex is determined by ethics, not biology (though once again I hasten to add that the contingencies of our bodies surely provide the material for that ethics; as the Marquis de Sade once commented, against the popular 'argument from design' that was circulating in natural theology': if God had not intended the anus to be used for sex he would not have shaped and positioned it so conveniently) [3].

5. SEXUAL PARADIGMS

I have by now, I hope, conveyed some sense of my thesis that our sexual conceptions are not wholly determined by the more mechanical contingencies of medical research. There is a logical and, more importantly, a cultural gap between functions and ideas, and it is more often the ideas that influence the functions rather than the other way around. (Even Marx and Engels would agree with this version of idealism, given that I have included most of the political and economic influences on the side of the 'ideas'.) Our conception of sex is to a certain extent centered on a paradigm, the two minute emissionary-missionary male-superior ejaculation service.

A paradigm need not be an ideal; indeed most paradigms tend to be boring examples, even in discussions of sex. But this paradigm has many facets, and so too draws upon many perspectives. In fact, heterosexual intercourse is not itself a paradigm so much as it is the convergence of many paradigms, and the job of a philosopher in addition to enjoying the practice, is to develop a theory in which these various paradigms are distinguished and played off against one another. There are four basic paradigms:

(1) the reproductive or procreative paradigm;
(2) the pleasure or 'recreational' paradigm;
(3) the metaphysical or 'Platonic' paradigm; and
(4) the intersubjective communication paradigm.

1.) The Reproductive Paradigm

The reproductive model has perhaps always been overemphasized, but, in the religious dress of 'procreation', it has been especially well-nourished under the auspices of the Christian church. It is a paradigm which distills off the pleasures and Romantic overtones of sex and reduces it to a matter of dutiful service to the species – or to God. The paradigm is typically embellished and not left in its cold biological state, but even so it is distinctively unconcerned with questions of mutual expression and tenderness. (The union of souls as well as bodies is a secondary development.) The paradigm of reproductive sexuality is the effective and efficient ejaculation of the male into the female. His orgasm is a bonus; hers is of no importance whatever. Indeed, excess enjoyment, wasting time and – most essentially – 'wasting seed', is perversion. Indeed, although the concept of 'perversion' did not really enter into sexual ethics and medicine until the 19th century, [6] the prohibitions against masturbation, sodomy, and all other manners of 'wasting seed' are found clearly even in the Old Testament. Needless to say, the sole paradigm here is heterosexual intercourse. Homosexuality has no place whatever, and even love and pleasure are at most of secondary importance as enticements, not telos.

Though nourished by religion, the reproductive model does not depend on religion for its persistence. Kant once argued that our sexual appetites are justified only insofar as they serve Nature's End, not our own. So too partisan politics or simple excessive biological conscientiousness can promote the reproductive paradigm. A Darwinian might see sex this way; a couple desperate to have children may temporarily conceive of their sexuality in this way, a sexual moralist might literally refer to 'natural sex' – in an argument against homosexuality for example – without invoking religion at any point. Indeed, this is often the more powerful and harder to refute version of moral arguments concerning sexuality, that our 'natural' desires are aimed at reproduction, whether consciously or not. 'Natural sex' is therefore sex aimed at reproduction, whether or not *we* aim at reproduction – or even thwart it – in our sexual activities. One might suggest, for instance, that such sex in general is 'practice' for the real thing, an odd suggestion which has, nevertheless, a considerable history behind it.

A paradigm is not necessarily an exclusive perspective, a set of blinders which permit only a single telos or conception. It is rather a matter of focus, a way of picking out certain features as essential and pushing others into the background. The reproductive paradigm highlights the biological consequences and minimizes the recreational and expressive features of sex. The procreational version of the paradigm adds to this the theology of divine design. Neither version need eliminate or ignore the other aspects of sexuality, but their emphasis already establishes an ethical framework. It is this framework within which the morals of contraception become heated issues, and it is within this framework that the technology of contraception has the greatest effect on our sexual conceptions. But there are other paradigms, and with them, other ethics and other concerns.

2.) The Pleasure Paradigm

The pleasure paradigm might be called 'liberal' as a reaction against the more conservative reproductive/procreative paradigm. It is, for the most part, the paradigm that provided the ideology of the sexual revolution of the 1960's and it is no coincidence that the most effective means of birth control ever invented coincided with this new ideology. But 'most effective' does not mean new or novel, and effectiveness is only one factor in the determination of sexual attitudes. Morals are often more effective than technological effectiveness or, in the case of the sexual revolution, some say the "lack of morals." Which is cause, which is effect? But here again we run up against that too simple-minded deterministic thesis. It is absurd to say that 'the pill' had nothing to do with the new attitude of freedom that defined the so-called 'revolution,' but it is equally nonsense to insist that it is by itself the cause of that cultural explosion. Contrary to traditional Freudian imagery, the 1960's were not the time of 'eros unchained' (one popular phrase of the period). There was not a massive libido suddenly released. Rather, there was a shift in paradigms, a swing of the Zeitgeist which included, not coincidentally, a new technology.

The real father of the sexual revolution is not Doctor Rock or Doctor Hertig but that ideologist of the libido, Sigmund Freud. It is Freud, for all of his personal sexual conservativism, who most soundly attacks the traditional reproductive/procreational paradigm and puts in its place a model of sex with pleasure as its telos and its defining characteristic [8]. Sex, for Freud, is not Nature's purpose, but rather the primary drive of the "psychic apparatus" to discharge itself. The pleasure paradigm, like the reproductive paradigm, rests on a biological foundation. It is the nervous system that is the locus of Freud's theory, and its physiological basis that determines the telos of sex. The goal of the nervous system, and of the organism, is Cartharsis, Freud tells us [7]. Its principle is homeostasis, or 'the constancy principle.' Its ultimate aim is emptiness and relaxation (a formulation that later led Freud into his flirtation with 'the Nirvana principle' and 'the death instinct'). The release of built-up tension is pleasure; the retention of tension is pain. The release or 'catharsis' of tension in sexuality produces the orgasm, and it is the pleasure of the orgasm – that is, the pleasure of release – that is the end of sexuality, not the procreative consequences of ejaculation. Thus it is important to note how central Freud's distinction between physical and psychic satisfaction becomes; it is the latter that is essential to successful sex, not the former. This simple picture is complicated by the fact that in addition to this 'primary process' there is a complex system of ego-needs, which involves identification with certain sexual 'objects.' Accordingly, sex becomes concerned with the satisfaction of these second-ary drives as well, and the simple pleasure of sex is complicated if not thwarted by the need for acceptance, security, and love. One might note the echo of Jean-Jacques Rousseau here, for Freud was also a "roman-tic" of sorts, but a pessimist à la Schopenhauer rather than a hopeful visionary like Rousseau. It is worth taking full note of the fact that, as release of tension, masturbation plays a central role in Freud's notion of sex, while in the reproductive paradigm this is at best a perversion, if not irrelevant to sex altogether.

The notion of 'discharge' or 'catharsis' in Freud's paradigm is obviously based on a male-oriented perspective. In this as well as in its biological foundation, it is not entirely distinct from the reproductive model. Understanding Freud, however, is not primarily a matter of the history of medicine so much as it is a socio-cultural concern; and his rebellion against the reproductive model is part and parcel of a far more general rebellion against a certain kind of society. So too, the pleasure model in its more modern version, whether the American Civil Liberties Union version which allows any sexual activity between 'mutually consenting adults,' or the more vulgar version that simply insists, 'if it feels good, do it', consists in part of a rebellion against restrictions no longer acceptable, paradigms no longer unchallengable. As a 'liberating' paradigm, the pleasure model needs no defense. A more difficult question is whether it is the best paradigm, a question that has become increasingly urgent in the counter-revolutionary years of the last decade.

What ails the pleasure paradigm? Fifteen years ago Rollo May wrote in a best-selling book, *Love and Will*, [11] that the sexual revolution has wrought its own forms of repression and unhappiness. His argument turns too much – in accord with that psychiatric genre – on the pathological, on the failures and victims of the revolution rather than its beneficiaries. Nevertheless, as both Freud and May warn us, with some justification, the plight of the neurotic may be a mirror – if a distorting mirror – of the pathology of everyday life. If the reproductive model makes sex too restrictive, the pleasure model makes it too conceptually permissive. Furthermore, any model of sexuality which makes masturbation as central or more central than intercourse, any model that refers to the other person in sexual desire as an 'object,' is an unlikely candidate for an adequate model of most of our sexual lives. Again, the paradigm may be liberating, but that does not mean that it is wholly adequate in itself.

Three main points of contention against the pleasure paradigm are the following:

(a) Aristotle argued 2500 years ago that pleasure is never the end of any of our activities, including sex [2]. It is rather the accompaniment of good activity, the enjoyment that comes from being virtuous and fulfilling one's telos. Thus the question becomes; What is the telos of sex that it gives us so much pleasure? What is it that we satisfy? What do we want? To say that pleasure is the *telos* of sex is to confuse the play with its musical accompaniment. (In that context, a consideration of the very different moods of making love, and the music that one might play along with them, is revealing.)

(b) Sex is mutual activity; masturbation, no matter how satisfying, is not our paradigm. At least part of the answer to the questions in (a) above is that there is satisfaction in being with or 'having' another person, not as a 'secondary' concern, as Freud has it, but as a primary concern. The promiscuity and lack of discrimination of aroused males aside, it is not an 'object' of sex we seek, but a partner.

(c) Moreover, because sex depends on concepts and paradigms as well as basic biology, our sexual behavior is never 'without' meaning.' Some meanings, however, are demeaning, and every sexual acts has its significance. To think that one can indulge in the traditionally most powerful symbolic activity in almost every culture without its meaning anything is an extravagant self-deception, which, nonetheless, does not prevent its wide-spread appearance in libertines and rakes of all ages.

3.) *The Metaphysical Paradigm*

The metaphysical paradigm is by far the most poetic of the four. We demand 'meaningful' relationships; this paradigm provides meaning. The metaphysical paradigm is Romantic love or eros; its classic text is Plato's *Symposium* [14] (thus I would also call it 'the Platonic paradigm', which is not to be conflated with the asexual notion of 'Platonic love' that emerged 15 centuries later). In simple-minded parlance, it is the vision that two people are 'made for each other.' Protestant Christianity often supplements or even replaces the procreative paradigm with this metaphysical paradigm, thus shifting the religious as well as the sexual emphasis to love *agape* not *eros*). The best picture of the metaphysical paradigm, however, is Aristophanes' wonderful tale in the *Symposium*, of a double creature cleft in two ('like an apple') by Zeus and ever since trying to find its 'other half' [14]. And indeed sex does sometimes seem like that, an experience so overwhelming and filled with significance that questions about the technology of contraception are not even plausible candidates for the defining features of our sexual conceptions.

4.) *The Intersubjective Paradigm*

The intersubjective or communication paradigm is the paradigm I would most like to defend, but I will not try to do so here. What I will do

SEX, CONTRACEPTION AND CONCEPTIONS OF SEX 239

here is offer it through an example, and then use it to conclude why it is that, in the course of my research, I have decided to minimize the seemingly obvious influence of sexual technology on sexual attitudes and concepts. The example comes from Jean-Paul Sartre [17]. For Sartre, unlike Freud, sex is essentially interpersonal. He does not deny that masturbation is sexual; there just is not anything very interesting to say about it. It is not just the consequences of sex that count; it is its meaning. But where the metaphysical paradigm tends to take a rather rosy view of meaning, Sartre sees quite clearly that meanings can be different. His dark vision is summarized in his famous play, *Huis Clos* (*No Exit*) [18]: 'Hell is other people.' Sex, accordingly, is essentially conflict, or, rather, it is the central battleground of our interpersonal wars. Sex is intersubjective: it is primarily concerned not with pregnancy or pleasure nor even togetherness, but rather with effecting as definitively as possible the other person's constitution of both him or herself, and oneself as well. It is a battle of domination and freedom, Sarte tells us. Sex, focuses the most inert parts of the body – breasts and buttocks. Not for pleasure and not for the sake of reproduction but, symbolically, Sartre says, 'to turn the other into an object,' to reduce him or her to a mere body in one's control. Every caress is manipulation; pleasure is an instrument, and one's own pleasure – far from being the goal of sex – may easily be a distraction and a defeat [17].

I do not endorse this gloomy view which, if taken whole, would put most of us in the land of the voluntary chaste. But its structure I consider nothing less than revolutionary – more revolutionary than even Freud's pleasure paradigm and the much touted sexual revolutions of the past. What Sartre does for us is to shift the paradigm once again, to sex as expression. It is not one's own pleasure that counts primarily (though one need not be indifferent to it) nor is it even the pleasure one produces in one's partner. Mutual pleasure production is not the telos of sex, even when, as so often, it is the most explicit focus of sex. (Kant, who died a virgin, once described sex as "mutual masturbation." [9]). One can correct Sartre's pessimistic picture by noting that love, too, is expressed through sex, but it is essential not to leap too quickly to the naive romanticism that says that only love is, or ought to be, expressed by sex. Sex is like a language, and there is no clear limit to the interpersonal feelings that it can express, given an adequate vocabulary and what we might call sexual literacy.

CONCLUSION: CONCEPTIONS AND CONCEPTION

My purpose here has been to demonstrate the conceptual complexity of a phenomenon too often viewed as primitive and uncomplicated, as if only the consequences are complications, not sex itself. I have shown that there is much more to sexuality than an enjoyable and occasionally productive biological process, and that the technology of sexual consequences – if I may call it that – is only part of, not the essential determinant of the nature of our sexual lives.

University of Texas at Austin
Austin, Texas

BIBLIOGRAPHY

1. Aristotle: 1943, *De Generatione Animalium*, translated by A. L. Peck, Harvard University Press, Cambridge.
2. Aristotle: 1925, *Nicomachean Ethics*, translated by W. D. Ross, Oxford University Press, Oxford.
3. de Sade, D.: 1965, *Justine, and Other Writings*, translated by R. Seaver and A. Wainhouse, Grove Press, New York.
4. Dover, K. J.: 1978, *Greek Homosexuality*, Harvard University Press, Cambridge.
5. Firestone, S.: 1970, *Dialectic of Sex*, William Morrow, New York.
6. Foucault, M.: 1978, *A History of Sexuality*, Vol. 1, Random House, New York.
7. Freud, S.: 1905, *Three Contributions to the Theory of Sex*, Dutton, New York.
8. Freud, S.: 1916, *Introductory Lectures on Psychoanalysis*, Hogarth Press, London.
9. Kant, I.: 1930, *Lectures on Ethics*, translated by L. Infield, Methuen, London, U.K.
10. Larkin, P.: 1974, "Annus Mirabilis", Farrar, Straus and Giroux, New York, N.Y.
11. May, R.: 1969, *Love and Will*, Norton, New York, N.Y.
12. Nietzsche, F.: 1974, *Gay Science*, transl. W. Kaufmann, Random House, New York, N.Y.
13. Nietzsche, F.: 1966, *Beyond Good and Evil*, transl. Walter Kaufmann, Random House, New York, N.Y.
14. Plato: 1892, *The Symposium*, translated by B. Jowett, Oxford University, Oxford, U.K.
15. Reed, J.: 1987, 'History of Contraceptive Practices', in this volume, pp. 15–38.
16. Rousseau, J.-J.: 1964, *Discourse on the Origins of Inequality*, transl. L. Crocker, Washington Square Press, New York, N.Y.
17. Sartre, J.-P.: 1943, *L'être et le Neant*, (*Being and Nothingness*), transl. H. Barnes, Philosophical Library, New York, N.Y.
18. Sartre, J.-P.: 1946, *Huis Clos* (*No Exit*), transl. S. Gilbert, Vintage Press, New York, N.Y.

STUART F. SPICKER

CONTRACEPTION AND CHANGING IMAGES OF SEXUALITY: COMMENTS ON MEREDITH MICHAELS' AND ROBERT SOLOMON'S REFLECTIONS

I

It is possible to offer two sets of comments here: a lengthy response to Professor Michaels' presentation and then on to Professor Solomon's essay – or a brief one. The brief one is as follows: To Michaels' question – "Is contraception a means of controlling one's personal destiny?" – she answers "No." To Solomon's question – "What rôle, if any, does contraception play in redefining sexuality of women and men?" – he answers "Virtually none." From the maxim, *ex nihilo nihil fit*, I could simply conclude in Wittgensteinian fashion – I could remain silent.

But I would be remiss in my duty to say nothing at all here, especially since, whereas Michaels and Solomon soar to the heavens and encounter destiny and the power of gods, I find myself confined here on non-picayune *terra firma*, embodied, bound by the life-world that is not infrequently independent of my actions, itself now astonishingly technological in the most complex and compelling ways; moreover, when I turn to the variety of traditional authorities for guidance, I find them all uncompelling. Encountering the gods, I usually discover Prometheus most enlightening and find myself the innocent recipient of his power. Recall the myth: Prometheus, who created man's body from water and clay and formed men in the likeness of gods, was judged arrogant by Zeus, who grew angry at man's increasing powers and talents. Thus Zeus withheld fire from mankind. But Prometheus, with assistance from Athene, stole away from Olympus, in possession of a glowing charcoal, undiscovered by Zeus, and, in time, gave fire to mankind ([1], pp. 34–35).

Accompanying Michaels' iteration of the grand myth of the power of the goddesses of destiny – Clotho, Lachesis and Atropos – who determined how long each mortal would live, which determined length even Zeus could not alter, there is the myth of Prometheus which portrays in vivid imagery the way mankind received the power of the gods in the form of fire. It is often overlooked that it was Athene who "breathed life into man's body" ([1], pp. 34–35), not Prometheus, for he only provided the material substance which would later be in-formed by Athene (in orthodox Aristotelian process metaphysics) as life itself.

241

Stuart F. Spicker, William B. Bondeson, and H. Tristram Engelhardt, Jr.
The Contraceptive Ethos, 241–248.

Thus Athene, a woman, is mother to us all. If it is the case, as Michael's suggests, that "contraception has been around as long as there have been people to tell about it . . ." ([2], p. 5), it is also a commonplace that motherhood was less problematic for the ancients than it turns out to be in our time. Before turning to the dialectical aspects of the contemporary technological advances which have made contraceptive practices rather significant in our time – I mean the *freedoms* engendered by pregnancy-avoidable sexual activity on the one hand and the paradoxical *inhibiting forces* weighing on desires of motherhood on the other – perhaps a word may be said to challenge the tacit and, at times, stated claim made by Michaels that contraceptive devices, since they were employed as early as 1900 B.C., reveal our world to be devoid of "creativity, progress, and originality in the field of contraceptive research . . ." ([2], pp. 4–5). For I also believe that we should avoid the 'historical and cultural myopia' of which Michaels warns, but I believe it equally important to underscore the clearly demonstrable truth of the proposition, *that with respect to the set of consequences which necessarily accompany heterosexual sexual activity and intercourse, the maximum negative consequences in our time are clearly less than ever before in history, whether Oriental or Occidental.* (If the reader doubts this assertion's truth, he or she could, as they say in the bar, 'Look it up'). In asserting this claim I do not intend to restrict the *consequences* to events like unwanted pregnancies, incurable venereal diseases, and some, though not all, earlier forms of contraception, but to speak of positive consequences of such human activity as longevity, healthier fetal and *ex utero* development of the infant, and perhaps motherhood (for many if not all women) as well as fatherhood.

II

Prior to the discussion, then, of the central issues raised by Professors Michaels and Solomon, it is worthwhile to distinguish, with the philosopher John Passmore, "ecological problems" from 'problems in ecology'. 'A problem in ecology', Passmore writes, "is a purely scientific problem, arising out of the fact that scientists do not understand some particular ecological phenomenon" ([3], p. 43). Hence, if we are interested in the ways, within our technological era, in which we can produce less and less, if not zero-risk contraceptive devices (whether chemical or mechanical, whether consumed by women or by men), any scientific solution will tend to bring us some understanding of the phenomena. In contrast, 'an ecological problem', Passmore continues, "is a special type of social problem" ([3], p. 43) and, moreover, we believe that our society would be better off without it. In the context of our concerns (the *Zeitgeist* dubbed by some "The Contraceptive Ethos"), the molar problem we would like to be rid of today is the very general one: people are pollution ([3], p. 127). Although this problem is not the principal one of this section of the volume, it is clearly related to earlier sections. That is, this ecological problem is simply that the world's population cannot continue to increase at its present rate;[1] the molecular form of this ecological problem of 'multiplication' with respect to individual decisions is the set of decisions to reproduce. (I believe that we have some consensus among the contributors to this volume that we shall not attend to the specific problems in ecology, the scientific problems, which are known to arise in the context of the molar ecological problem of overpopulation, that is, the empirical problems of 'how to' produce less and less risky contraceptive substances and devices to protect ourselves from unwanted pregnancies, even the curable venereal diseases, and other apparently dire consequences of our sexual encounters. More-over, I leave out here the newest actor on the stage of infirmity which epidemiologists will explore at a later date when they do retrospective studies on the AIDS and Herpes epidemics in all their virulent variants. At the present time, the important empirical questions focus on the development and production of a zero-risk, mechanical device which can be safely (and non-surgically) inserted into the woman's Fallopian tubes until such time as she decides to plan to become pregnant.[2] Until then, however, we shall continue to concern ourselves with the risks attendant to various forms of steroid hormones ('the pill'), intra-uterine devices (IUDs), barrier devices, vaginal and other more-recently developed spermicides, postcoital douches, and even the non-chemical *coitus interruptus* (as if saying it in Latin makes it any less frustrating and psychologically inert). We must, of course, not lose sight of the fact that in spite of living on the historical edge of the contraceptive ethos, which Michaels and Solomon have assailed for its lack of profundity and impact on our lives (with some justification, of course), there are and have been other more radical methods employed to control the phenomenon of multiplication which, in our time, is over, not underpopulation.

That is, we should also mention, along with the various contraceptive devices (including Professor Reed's reference to "divorce" and other forms of contraception which are equally unappealing to our sensibilities), periodic abstinence or total continence (celibacy) from sexual intercourse, sterilization in its various surgical and non-surgical forms, abortion, in its various modalities, infanticide, the imposition of legal and/or economic enactments and sanctions and, of course, the so-called 'natural' phenomena of war, pestilence and epidemics (hardly 'natural' at all, given Solomon's firm blow to this oft-misused notion).

With these initial remarks, I turn to the central issues raised by Michaels and Solomon.

First, both philosophers focus their attention on the complex relation that obtains between contraception (including its technological forms) *and* both sexual and reproductive freedom ([2], p. 2; [5], p. 11); they both seem to agree that notwithstanding the more technologically advanced forms of contraception now available, the inference that we are today more free or sexually liberated is more myth than reality. Michaels goes a step further: There is no new freedom in fact, for "individual liberty can [not] emerge independent of social and economic constraints" ([2], p. 9). I believe Solomon, too, agrees with this claim ([5], p. 17). Both Michaels and Solomon avoid dwelling, as many do, on the separation between sexual activity via contraception not aimed at reproduction *and* the specific reproductive aims of some, though not all, sexual activity ([2], p. 5). (With the advent of *in vitro* fertilization and embryo transfer, by the way, we now have achieved the final break indeed – reproduction without sexual intercourse.) In short, Michaels concludes that although reproductive freedom is 'currently enjoyed by women' it is conditional "but is not truly in their hands" ([2], p. 10). To support her assertion, Michaels distinguishes (1) the fact that reproduction decisions *can* with assurance today be carried out thanks to contraceptive devices of various kinds, from (2) the decision to *actually use* any of these methods to avoid or delay pregnancy, or even to achieve it in order to assume the rôle of mother ([2], pp. 12, 19). I take it that the second is truly reproductive freedom in Michael's view. Hence she, having made this distinction, can say that she in no way wishes "to underestimate the crucial role played by contraception in establishing reproductive choice". What troubles her is that the decision to use or not use contraceptives does not entail the decision to be a mother. What we witness here, then, is neither an inappropriate nor a trivial distinction; but what is puzzling, indeed, is Michaels' suggestion that anyone would have thought that having the option to use accessible, inexpensive, efficient, safe and openly-dispensed and discussed contraceptives would have any bearing whatsover on the rôle (not to mention the narrative) of motherhood. That is, the dilemma which she poses is that either one choses to become pregnant or one does not. If a woman does and bears a child, she fails; if she avoids this outcome she fails as a woman. The notion that she fails in either case is interesting, but misleading. The point to underscore, it seems to me, is that during the time or times a woman is trying (perhaps struggling) to determine whether or not to become pregnant and have a child she is quite free, in one sense of freedom, to enjoy her sexual life (perhaps not now construed in relation to reproduction) as only she, without the voices of external authority, dictates.

Professor Solomon, who elects to leave the discussion of biologic conception aside ([5], p. 3), focuses his attention on sexual conceptions (conceptions of sex) and the meaning of 'sex'. He holds that contraception has not altered our notion of sex, nor freed us from 'extraneous fears' ([5], p. 1). But he also says in the end (but only *at* the end) that the 'technology of sexual consequences' e.g., contraception and unwanted pregnancy, is "a part of, not the essential determinant of, the nature of our sexual lives" ([5], p. 38). What I have suggested thus far applies here as well: This 'part' that contraceptive technology plays is in need of further exploration. That is, it is a gross simplification to conclude that our sexual conceptions have not been dramatically affected and determined by contraceptive technology, biomedicine, and the cure and prevention of various sexually transmitted diseases; moreover, we ought not to leave the issue of our 'attitudes toward contraception' unaddressed ([5], p. 13). Put another way, if it is the case that our attitudes toward sexuality determine our interests in contraception, as Solomon maintains, there is no reason to think the inversion empty and without any truth: Namely, that the advent of modern forms of contraception (and forms yet to be perfected which will prove virtually risk free, even more affordable, efficient, and accessible for use in a sexually open society) will have a profound effect and dramatic bearing on our attitudes toward sexuality – on our own embodiment, its indwelling in freedom, its confidence, and its comfort and pleasure.

III

In closing, I shall take up one additional matter: Solomon's attack on the *libertarian paradigm*. I need not repeat his description of this and the other paradigms he mentions [4], but he does say that the libertarian paradigm is 'too simple-minded' ([5], p. 21). This, it seems to me, is in need of some analysis and argument. Clearly, Solomon appeals to the *absence* of 'mutuality of expression' in this paradigm, but I fail to see why the libertarian view, which is not intrinsically licentious, is incompatible with such mutuality ([5], p. 25). And why does he say it is 'too conceptually permissive'? ([5], p. 24) Is there some human telos at work, that holding such a view, does not permit those holding it to fulfill? How, in short, does this view block the 'infinite yearning' ([5], pp. 9, 14) which Solomon seems to value? Quite the contrary: Does not this view finally permit us to freely construe our bodies as under our control at last? In this context, remember, it is not the fire stolen by Prometheus, in the modern form of technology that is our unrequested burden, but the awesome responsibility for ourselves, our precious sexuality, and our personal destiny, which is so personal in fact that Sartre could say that we are 'condemned to be free'. Nothing makes this clearer than the impetus of the contraceptive ethos that is, historically speaking, quite new and has led some, I think, to under-estimate the significance of its power to transform the very relation we have (or shall soon have) with our own embodiment in all its richness. Here I can only offer a suggestion, a metaphor perhaps: There was a time when the Ptolemaic cosmology predominated, the earth was conceived as flat, and the stars known to move daily across the heavens. The sun used to rise and set. Such a world, since the Copernican revolution, is more and more an illusion. Today the Copernican cosmology is so all-pervasive that the youngest school child can virtually prove Ptolemy in error, and his own father a fool for suggesting that the earth is solid under him, the sun about to rise, the stars in motion overhead at dusk and evening. Do you get my drift? A most powerful cosmology can, over decades and centuries, find its way into the very conception we have of ourselves; so, too, our new conception of controlled conception via contraception will, in the not too distant future, be shown to have had equal power over us all. In this claim I simply repeat Solomon's notion that "Sex is ideas", but I take it – and if space permitted would carry it – all the phenomeological way. But since we are only at the edge of the contraceptive ethos of which I speak, we cannot be faulted, really, for tending to take lightly the very recent technological advances which enable Solomon to say, with respect to heterosexual intercourse, that it is now possible to have it succeeded by sleep (television on or off) rather than by unwanted pregnancy followed by abortion or birth ([5], p. 16).

The myth of Prometheus suggests that some new power is now at work, which has, at the very least, been transferred to our hands if not our brains. Is the acceptance of this transmutation of power and responsibility not precisely the precondition for the partial realization of that 'infinite yearning' as expressed in our embodied sexuality? Why, then, is the libertarian paradigm any less devoid of symbolic significance? ([5], p. 25) Does not this paradigm possess all the necessary ingredients to qualify as at one with what Solomon calls the "positive comunication" paradigm? Are sexual desire, sex, and sexual activity any less *sex as expression*? Perhaps I am asking for too much, for Solomon explicitly concludes his essay by saying that although "he would most like to defend" this view of Aristophanes, he does not wish to do so here. I sincerely hope he does so *somewhere*, for I, for one, would like to be privy to those reflections. Until that time, however, I think it perfectly good for each superwoman and superman to swive on the brink of the abyss, for even there they can do so in tenderness, if not always in love.

The University of Connecticut,
School of Medicine
Farmington, Connecticut

NOTES

[1] According to the authors of [6], "By the year 2000, the world's population is projected to increase by between 1.5 billion and 2.1 billion people" ([6], p. iii) They continue: "Rapidly declining death rates combined with continuing high birth rates are producing unprecedented world population growth, some 92% of which is occurring in less developed countries (LDCs). . . . The current world population of 4.4 billion is projected to reach about 6.2 billion (range: 5.9 billion to 6.5 billion) in 2000. Eighty million people are being added to the world annually; this number is expected to rise to 95 million per year by 2000 (range: 70 million to 120 million)" ([6], pp. 29, 163).

[2] A very promising method of sterilization for women (Hysteroscopic Tubal Occlusion with Silicone Rubber, or Oviduct Blocking with Formed-in-Place Silicone Rubber Plugs) has been reported in the medical literature by Drs. Theodore P. Reed and Robert A. Erb. The physicians do not claim, at this time, that this new method of non-surgical (and non pharmacologic) tubal sterilization is, if reversible, the 'solution' for the search for the optimum, safe, and effective form of contraception. The technique involves "the flowing of catalyzed silicone material into the oviduct through a silicone rubber obturator tip positioned at the tubal ostium." (See Erb, R. A. and Reed, T. P.: 1979, 'Hysteroscopic Oviductal Blocking with Formed-in-Place Silicone Rubber Plugs: I. Method and Apparatus', *Journal of Reproductive Medicine*, **23** (2), 65). It should be noted that the researchers do remark that: "The potential exists for it to become one of the leading methods of

contraception and a valuable new tool in family plannuing" (*Ibid.*, p. 68). Also see, *Ibid.*; II. Clinical Studies' 69–72; Reed, T. P. Erb, R. A., and DeMaeyer, J.: 1981, 'Tubal Occlusion with Silicone Rubber: Update, 1980', *Journal of Reproductive Medicine* **26** (10), 534–537; and Reed, T.P. and Erb, R.: 'Hysteroscopic Tubal Occlusion with Silicone Rubber', *Obstetrics & Gynecology* **61** (3), 388–392.

BIBLIOGRAPHY

1. Graves, R.: 1955, *The Greek Myths: Volume I*, Chapter 39, Penguin Books, Middlesex, U.K.
2. Michaels, M. W.: 1987, 'Contraception, Freedom and Destiny: A Womb of One's Own', in this volume, pp. 207–219.
3. Passmore, J.: 1974, *Man's Responsibility for Nature: Ecological Problems and Western Traditions*, Charles Scribner's Sons, New York, N.Y.
4. Solomon, R. C.: 1974, 'Sexual Paradigms', *Journal of Philosophy* **71** (11), 336–345.
5. Solomon, R. C.: 1987, 'Sex, Conception and Conceptions of Sex', in this volume, pp. 221–238.
6. U.S. Government Printing Office: 1982, *World Population and Fertility Planning Technologies: The Next 20 Years*, Office of Technology Assessment, L.C.C. No. 82–600516, Washington, D.C.

NOTES ON CONTRIBUTORS

William B. Bondeson, Ph.D., is Professor of Philosophy, Department of Philosophy, University of Missouri–Columbia, Columbia, Missouri.

Nancy Neveloff Dubler, LL.B., is Director, Division of Legal and Ethical Issues in Health Care, Department of Social Medicine, Montefiore Hospital and Medical Center, The Bronx, New York.

H. Tristram Engelhardt, Jr., Ph.D., M.D., is Professor of Medicine and of Community Medicine, and Member, Center for Ethics, Medicine and Public Issues, Baylor College of Medicine, Houston, Texas.

Thomas Halper, Ph.D., is Professor and Chairman, Department of Political Science, Baruch College and The Graduate Center, City University of New York, New York.

Jonathan Lieberson, Ph.D., is an Associate, Center for Policy Studies, The Population Council, New York, and Visiting Professor, Barnard College, New York.

Meredith W. Michaels, Ph.D., is Assistant Professor of Philosophy, Department of Philosophy, Hampshire College, Amherst, Massachusetts.

Constance A. Nathanson, Ph.D., is Professor, Department of Population Dynamics, School of Hygiene and Public Health, The Johns Hopkins University, Baltimore, Maryland.

The Honorable John T. Noonan, Jr.. J. D., is United States Circuit Judge, Ninth Circuit Court of Appeals, and Milo Robbins, Professor of Law, Emeritus, University of California School of Law, 464 Boalt Hall, Berkeley, California.

James Reed, Ph.D., is Professor of History, Department of History, Rutgers University, New Brunswick, New Jersey.

Janet W. Salaff, Ph.D., is Professor of Sociology, Department of Sociology, University of Toronto, Ontario, Canada.

Hans-Martin Sass, Ph.D., is Visiting Scholar, The Kennedy Institute of Ethics, Center for Bioethics, Georgetown University, Washington, D.C. and Professor of Philosophy, Institut für Philosophie, Ruhr-Universität Bochum, Bochum-Querenburg, West Germany.

Robert C. Solomon, Ph.D., is Professor of Philosophy, Department of Philosophy, University of Texas at Austin, Austin, Texas.

Stuart F. Spicker, Ph.D., is Professor of Community Medicine and Health Care (philosophy), School of Medicine, University of Connecticut Health Center, Farmington, Connecticut.

INDEX

The Philosophy and Medicine Book Series

Editors

H. Tristram Engelhardt, Jr. and Stuart F. Spicker